eating wisely for hormonal balance

The Woman's Guide to Good Health, High Energy & Ideal Weight

SONIA GAEMI, ED.D., RD

New Harbinger Publications, Inc.

Dedication

Eating wisely starts in mothers' wombs. World healing starts with self-healing.

To my grandchildren, Sophia, Koosha, Leila, Kian, Sasha, Denna, and all the other seeds of our future planet.

To my energy healing Chinese medicine qigong masters, colleagues, and to my contributing teachers: my students and my friends. This book also is dedicated to all women who have bridged Eastern wisdom and Western science to achieve hormonal balance. When women's wisdom is heard, the world will be healed.

Distributed in Canada by Raincoast Books.

Copyright © 2004 by Sonia Gaemi
New Harbinger Publications, Inc.
5674 Shattuck Avenue
Oakland, CA 94609

Cover design by Amy Shoup
Interior images by PhotoDisc, Brand X Pictures, and Stockbyte
Cover photo by Morgan Karami

ISBN 1-57224-373-2 Paperback

Printed in the United States of America

New Harbinger Publications' Web site address: www.newharbinger.com

06   05   04

10   9   8   7   6   5   4   3   2   1

First printing

Contents

Acknowledgments   vii

Preface   ix
Food for Hormonal Healing * Learning from the Past * The
Wisdom of Stories * My Background * Four Things to Remember

Introduction to Food Wisdom   I
Eat for Health and Pleasure * A Revolution in Health Is
Needed * Wise Eating for a Balanced Life * Who Else Can Benefit
from This Book * Scientific Research * Alkalinity and Acidity * The
Food Wisdom Pyramid * Balance Your Health with the Pyramid
* The Pyramid Ways * The Food Wisdom Model * Food Wisdom
Goals

chapter 1
How Your Hormones Work   15
Food and Your Hormones * The Role of Estrogen and Progesterone
* Your Personal Health Concerns * Women's Need for Balanced
Hormones * Hormonal Eating Is a Lifelong Process * Eating Wisely
for Hormonal Balance * Trans-Fatty Acids and Saturated Fat * Food
Wisdom for Menopause * Healthy Hearts for Women * Lowering
Blood Pressure with Heart Friendly Foods * Foods for Strong
Bones * Integrating East and West for Body, Mind, and Spirit

chapter 2

Food Wisdom for Life 41

Making the Kitchen the Center of Busy Lives * Keeping a Food Diary * Recording Methods * You Can Diagnose Problems * Realize Your Food Wisdom Goals * Your Kitchen: The Heart of Your Home. * Food Wisdom Planning Goals * A Wise Shopping List

chapter 3

The Cleansing Way for Energy and Health 60

Spring for Your Body and Mind * The Cleansing Way * Spiced Leafy Greens, Sprouts, and Fruits * Shopping and Preparing for Cleansing * Consider a Blender * The Cleansing Plans * Food Sensitivities * A Few Favorites

chapter 4

The Morning Way 77

The First Food of the Day * Fiber Breakfast for Healthy Digestion and Daylong Energy * A Colorful Rainbow of Phytochemicals * Plant Protein for Bright Mornings and Alert Days * Variety through Grains * Root Vegetables * Putting Your Morning Way Plan into Action

chapter 5

Tea, Oxygen, and Movement 94

Tea: Bridging East and West * Cultural Wisdom about Every Breath You Take * Move through Your Life for Fitness and Fun

chapter 6

Snacking Your Way to Good Health 111

Wise Snacking * Learn to Snack on Healthy Food * The American Way of Snacking * The Positive Value of Snacking * Snacking to Satisfy Your Basic Urges * Eat Low Glycemic Foods for Steady Energy * Mother Nature's Bountiful Plant Foods * Indulge Your Senses with Healthy Choices * Snack Foods and Fat * Salt: How Much Is Too Much? * Setting Goals

chapter 7

Healthy Weight and Healthy Hormones   126

Healthy Weight * Use the Food You Eat * Weight Gain during
Midlife * Underweight or Overweight: Both Are Problems * The
Role of the Food Industry * How You Look at It * Taking Control
of Your Weight * The Glycemic Index and Weight Control * Insulin
Resistance and Chromium * Insulin and Serotonin, the Mood
Hormones * Foods That Help Manage Diabetes * Calcium and
Weight * Tips for Maintaining a Healthy Weight * Your Thyroid
Gland's Power over Weight, Life, and Death * Food Wisdom for a
Healthy Weight

chapter 8

Preventing and Relieving Major Symptoms of   147
Hormonal Imbalances

Food Wisdom Prescriptions * Allergies or Food Sensitivities *
Anemia and Fatigue * Arthritis or Osteoarthritis * Constipation
and Irregularity * Diabetes * Diarrhea * Gastrointestinal Problems
* Premenstrual Syndrome * Headaches and Migraines * Cancer
Recovery and Support * Hair Loss * Heart Problems * High
Blood Pressure * Complications from Hysterectomy * Hot Flashes
or Sweating * Insomnia * Symptoms Associated with Menopause *
Osteoporosis

chapter 9

The Joy of Herbs and Spices   171

Spices and Herbs, Blended into Your Life * Relearning the
Wisdom of Herbs and Spices * Spice and Herb Tips * The
Art of Flavoring with Herbs and Spices

chapter 10

Recipes for Balanced Hormones   183

The Basics * Morning Way Recipes * Salads and Greens *
Soups * Fish * Snacks * Sweet Things

References   205

Acknowledgments

Thank you to the 5,000 women around the world who shared their food and energy healing wisdom with me and helped me give birth to this book. They taught me ancient wisdom from the Persian Empire to the Silk & Spices Road, from China's wall to Chinese traditional medicinal Qi Gong, and shared Rumi's healing with love.

Mary Rudge, Jean Shinoda Bolen, professor Hui Liu, Grandmaster Yang Moi Jun, Dr. Jun-Ann Clark, and Dr. Sheldon Margen support me in my efforts to bring to the women of the globe the leadership lesson of the wild geese, to open our wings to the world and to look at the earth as a child to be nurtured and as a mother to nurture. From the mothers' wombs, to men and women all over the planet, we bring the seeds of wise eating.

Brazilian revolutionary, philosopher, and educator Paolo Freire showed us that the foundation of education is to teach people to teach themselves. *Eating Wisely for Hormonal Balance* is based on the idea that the way to self-healing and world healing begins with women's wisdom and leadership. The wisdom of my teachers, colleagues, and friends will live on in my work on the first women's satellite TV show in the world, in the healing centers I help to set up all over the world, and in my work with the Institute of Women's Cultural Wisdom (WCW).

I must also thank Dr. Sheldon Margen and Dale Ogar, Dr. Erlene Chiang, Susan J. Zipp, Ann Coulston, Dr. Anansa Taharka, Lynn Twist, Master Sha, Dr. Deepak Chopra, Leanne Backer, Foojan Zieni, Shirley Dean, Tom Bates, Karola Saekel, Dr. Sadja Greenwood, Dana and Peter Christy, Sharzad Ardelan, Helen Yee, Lida Kompanian, Arjang Zendehdel, Dr. Noman Narchi, Parnian Kaboli, Judy Timmel, Donna Sofaer, Reb Anderson, Mel Sujan, Christy Kimbra, Dr. Beverly Rubik, Dr. Effie Chow, Dr. Katherin Smith, Dr. Kristin Van De Carr, Dr. Doddy Messersmith, Dr. Ronda Tycer, Dr. Kenneth Fan, Justin Toal, Andrea Nasser and Sholeh Hamedani, Diane Valentine, Dr. Marti Lee Kenneday, Tomoko Lipp, Joyce Gerter, and Virginia Mejia, Heather Hutcheson, Connie Chan Robinson, Christine Shuk Yin Yu, Rachel Kranz, Parman Kublie, Anita and Al Rosso, Helen Yee, David and Solie Hashemi, Wes Nicker, Dr. Mary Lee, Diane Littlefield of Women's Health Leadership, Carol Hansen Grey, Gathering The Women, United Nation USA/Berkeley and Mytherapynet.com.

Thank you to my husband, Ghassem, my son Nasser and his wife Mindy, my daughter Katosha and her husband Afshin, and to my grandchildren.

My editor, Melissa Kirk, acted as my soul, patiently and quietly honoring my passion to give birth to this book. Without everyone at New Harbinger Publications who worked so hard on this project, I couldn't have opened my wings and brought this book to the planet.

To everyone else who has inspired me with their love, wisdom, and strength, you are all in my heart.

Preface

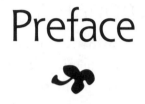

I have always loved food. I have made my home in different regions of the world, and everywhere I have lived or visited I have fallen in love with the flavors, spices, and aromas of new foods, with their color, beauty, and textures, and with their luscious abundance of tastes.

As a young girl, I asked my mother and grandmother their secrets—what they put in the dishes they served to their friends, the foods that people raved over and couldn't get enough of. My father, too, loved the art of cooking and sharing food, and people considered him a great chef. I was often with him in our herb garden and the kitchen, watching and learning.

My grandparents and parents emigrated from Russia to the Middle East and Iran, where I was born. My parents believed in celebrating with food and sharing ideas about the power of healing with food; in my family, eating was the most pleasant of pastimes. True, food was a necessity, but we were also excited about food.

Throughout my life, I have relished meals shared with friends and family and have enjoyed experimenting with food preparation. I have watched women of various cultures as they ate, fed young children, and let young people learn with them. Instinctively and from centuries of tradition, they understood how certain foods nourished the body. They sipped many kinds of teas and ate herbs to avoid menstrual cramps, to overcome a head cold, to increase their energy, to relax, to aid digestion, and to have a good sleep. My passion was to learn this wisdom of food. ❧

food for hormonal healing

Hormonal eating means eating foods that support your hormonal needs and all of your nutrition needs, helping you maintain a balanced weight and a healthy metabolism through all stages of your life.

In the West, a lucrative business has evolved, claiming to correct hormonal imbalances in women. Hormone pills and patches may do more harm than good to women's bodies, and a Western lifestyle of eating, including the consumption of processed foods, may cause many health problems attributed to aging.

Anti-aging in America has involved surgical and other methods to reshape and remove flesh and skin, while in many other countries women rejuvenate their cells, change their weight and appearance, and balance their hormones with combinations of natural whole food plants.

In Western society, specialists tend to treat parts of the body, not the whole person, and look more to technological solutions through medications made from plant parts and engineered plants, It is best to use parts of the actual plant rather than to take synthetic supplements and laboratory-created medicines, because there are many components within plants that help the body stay healthy, some of which are not yet understood by modern medicine. ❧

learning from the past

The Egyptians and people of the Mediterranean, Middle East, and Asia, as well as in South and Central America, created the first pyramids—the same design that is used in food pyramids today. Though each came independently to the design, so far as we know today, all were united in believing that this structure was created for the purpose of holding the body safe from decay. Pyramids support the spirit's eternal and individual creative journey. ❧

the wisdom of stories

I've included many of examples of food wisdom success stories from my e-mail correspondence, workshops, clients, international cable T.V. show, and students, and from interviews I've conducted. These stories tell of the interesting and often unrealized conditions that food imbalances cause and what changes women have made in their attitude toward food and their experiences with food for healing.

I've also included information about food and recipes from many cultures. You will learn some ancient food secrets and discover the variety of foods women all over the world enjoy. My goal, the goal of food wisdom, is to teach you to savor the magnificent feast offered by Mother Nature and to learn to work with your lifestyle and food choices to staying young, relaxed, and joyful. ❧

my background

I have enjoyed more than thirty years studying and researching the effects of nutrition and various foods through the body-mind connection while working as a mother, home chef, television producer and host, journalist, Chinese medicine and qigong instructor, nutritionist, registered dietitian, researcher, and food therapist with a multicultural focus. This book includes the wisdom of people from the Middle East, Canada, Russia, Australia, Africa, the Mediterranean, and Latin America, as well as Hispanics, Asians, African-Americans, and Caucasians in their countries of origin, and in the multiethnic United States. I have studied women's lifestyles, their common beliefs, the foods they eat, food celebrations and rituals, as well as their health concerns, healing arts, and nutrition. ❧

four things to remember

I want you to know as much as possible about

- Hormones: How they affect our sense of physical and mental well-being, as well as our health.

- A hormonal diet: How our diets can make an enormous difference to our metabolism and hormonal balance.

- Food wisdom: How women around the world have used their traditional food wisdom to resolve and prevent their hormonal problems—an approach that is finally available to U.S. women.

- How to spice up your diet: Women can easily add greens, herbs, spices, nuts, seeds, and teas to their current diets, with surprisingly good results!

Throughout this book, you will learn to design your own step-by-step approach to food wisdom that will help you make healthy changes as you listen to your body, instincts, and senses.

Introduction to Food Wisdom

Aging is wisdom, and is a natural path to important insight.
—Dr. Sadja Greenwood, MD

everyone must eat to live. Food has a potent influence on your well-being. The latest scientific research confirms what most people already know: no matter what supplements you take, no matter how much you exercise, no matter what health program you are on, you will not be healthy unless you eat a balance of healthy, energizing foods. Studies show that unhealthy eating habits can bring on hormone imbalances, allergies, asthma, high blood pressure, PMS and menopause symptoms, arthritic pain, leg cramps, weight problems, cravings, diabetes, and other health problems.

Yet, just as food can cause health problems, it can also help address them. Since we must eat anyway, why not find appealing ways to use food to balance and extend our life happily?

My approach to food will complement any other health plan you may be on. It offers advice for women of all ages, from teens to women of child-bearing age, to perimenopausal, menopausal, and postmenopausal women. The body should feel healthy. Being a woman is not a disease, and women's bodies exist for their happiness, health, and beauty. ❧

eat for health & pleasure

Many people think the word *diet* symbolizes loss or food restriction. The word comes from the Greek root *diatia* and the Latin *diaeta*, which mean "to live one's life" and "manner of living," respectively. Diet encompasses your total lifestyle. Your food choices should enhance your ability to live life fully—and not cause you to feel hungry, deprived, fatigued, or ill. Your eating style should be generous, open, and all encompassing. My food wisdom therapy for women, with the food wisdom pyramid that I'll introduce shortly as its model, can be bountiful, glorious, enjoyable, and delicious.

The goal of this book is to help women learn how they can benefit from *phytohormonals* (compounds found in plants that have hormonelike effects), antioxidants, and other nutrients found in food by making good dietary choices. Each culture has its own foods strong in fiber and phytohormones, foods enjoyed for their unique flavors and traditional tastes. Science is learning that these foods often have protective health benefits. Many of these benefits are directly related to changes in the body caused by hormone fluctuation.

We now know that eating the right foods may save our lives. People live longer and healthier lives in some cultures; now studies show that what these people eat is a factor. In studying the diets of cultures with lower rates of cancer, osteoporosis, heart disease, and obesity, many medical researchers have found their diets to be naturally abundant in fiber and phytohormonal foods, balanced with a variety of whole foods. ❧

a revolution in health is needed

Today, we're seeing the results of a steady diet high in protein, fats, calories, and technologically developed foods, such as Nutrasweet and Olestra. High-stress jobs, few or no regular healthy activities, and consumption of overprocessed foods with too many artificial food additives and many refined, denatured, diet foods all contribute to the high incidence of chronic illnesses in our society. I have known people to eat themselves sick and over time eat themselves to death.

In countries like America, salt, sugar, and fat permeate snack choices and can lead to insulin imbalances which may cause mood swings, feelings of stress, fatigue, and obesity, even among children. The chemical substances in salt, sugar, and fats and the quantity and quality of some fats that have become popular adversely affect the hormones. 🍀

wise eating for a balanced life

As you assess your hormonal condition consider if you have sleeplessness, tension, and stress from a busy lifestyle; if you are a mother hoping to prevent disease and raise healthy children; if you have been treated for breast cancer or are receiving other treatments affecting your immune system; or if you have other health concerns. I have written out easy ways for you to plan quick meals for balanced nutrition.

No matter what you enjoy eating or how you presently think about the food you eat, the cultural wisdom about food gathered here will teach you how and why to make choices from Mother Nature's bounty. I present new food combinations, cooking techniques, and information about the foods you love, as well as some you may not have tried because they seemed too difficult to prepare.

You will read, perhaps for the first time, about how hormone imbalances can affect your body's functioning. Foods that support female hormones are explained in depth, with chapters devoted to your complex body system. Food wisdom offers a balanced approach to the body and its workings, explaining how certain foods can be used therapeutically for wellness, to improve and maintain health, and to heal the body and mind. ❧

who else can benefit from this book

In addition to helping individuals, this book also may serve

- doctors or practitioners looking to encourage healthy eating habits in their patients;

- HMOs seeking preventive approaches to disease;

- nutritionists, nurses, physicians' assistants, midwives, chiropractors, homeopaths, naturopathic doctors, and many other alternative, traditional, and holistic healers, all of whom understand that a healthy diet supports other types of healing and prevention;

- retreat and resort centers, schools, women's groups, and other institutions concerned about women's health and well-being.

Remeber that following food wisdom therapy should help your well-being and may help with specific medical conditions, but it is not a substitute for appropriate medical care. Be sure to talk over ideas and information regarding food wisdom therapy with medical professionals if you have a serious medical condition or are taking doctor-prescribed medications regularly. ❧

scientific research

Based on research done in the fields of phytohormonals, fiber, and anti-oxidants, this book shows ways in which colors, flavors, and textures of food can affect your health and well-being. You'll also learn to enhance your food with flavorful spices that may strengthen your immune system and help you remain energetic and strong.

We need a wide variety of foods in our diets, partly because each of our organs is supported by different-colored foods. You will become a food artist, seeing the colorful food on your plate in a whole new way, supporting your brain, skin, heart, energy, even mood, by the chemistry in the colors you choose. ❧

alkalinity & acidity

Food has qualities that are either alkaline or acidic. In Eastern cultures, these qualities are called yin and yang, in the Middle East, *sardi* and *garmi*, and in Western society they are known as foods that supply essential heat or coolness throughout the body. In my practice, I have observed specific health problems that relate to the balance of foods and have discovered that many of these problems can be treated by changing the diet in favor of acidic food if alkalinity is a problem or vice versa.

Another food quality is its glycemic index, which affects hormones, weight, and metabolism. The glycemic qualities of foods are covered in chapter 7.

Typical alkaline, or yin, foods include: barley, beef, bread, butter, cabbage, cauliflower, celery, cherries, citrus fruits, cranberries, cucumber, eggplant, fish (except for snapper), grapefruit, green beans, kidney beans, lettuce, peaches, peas, peanuts, pinto beans, rice, spinach, strawberries, tomato, turnip, water chestnuts, anise, cilantro, green apples, lentils, mint, mung beans, pears, plum, pomegranate, prunes, pumpkins, rhubarb, spinach, watermelon, yogurt, coriander, dill, mint.

Typical acidic, or yang, foods include: red apple, banana, buckwheat, cantaloupe, carrot, cashews, cheese, chocolate, poultry, dates, eggs, garbanzo beans, grapes, honey, green pepper, honeydew melon, lamb, leeks, mangos, millet, black mushrooms, okra, pecans, persimmon, pistachio, pork, raisins, red snapper, sprouted beans and seeds, sweet potatoes, walnuts, wheat, yellow split peas, angelica, basil, bay leaves, black pepper, cardamom, celery seed, chamomile, chile peppers, chives, cinnamon, cloves, cumin seed, curry powder, fennel, fenugreek, ginger, garlic, lemon grass, licorice, marjoram, nutmeg, onion, parsley, rose, saffron, salt, shallots, tarragon, turmeric, vanilla, vinegar.

Neutral foods include: brown rice, corn, soybeans, oats, sunflower seeds, Brazil nuts, most dried beans and peas, tofu, almonds, olive oil, flax seeds, white mushrooms, tea, unsalted feta cheese. ❧

the food wisdom pyramid

The pyramid created by the United States Department of Agriculture (USDA) and seen on food packages throughout the United States was revolutionary when it was introduced in 1992 because it brought about a healthy emphasis on grains and protein.

My belief is that the food groups of the USDA model don't go far enough to explore food diversity and foods that are therapeutic and healing for women. The pyramid has been widely criticized and the USDA is currently revising it.

Most research done in the Western world has been on men's health, and the standard pyramids used today have been based on these studies. Along with members of many international health associations with whom I have worked in my nutrition studies, I wanted a way to help women of all ages achieve better health and prevent diseases in an economical, easy, and universally applicable way. And so, my food wisdom pyramid is designed especially for women's unique needs. As you can see from the figure on the next page, I have turned the standard pyramid upside down to ask you to think differently about food. By turning the pyramid on its point, I hope you will remember the most important aspect of any good diet: balance. This food wisdom pyramid will help you maintain good health by balancing all your bodily functions.

In developing a new pyramid, I took the latest principles of nutrition science advocated by leading U.S. health organizations and added

The Food Wisdom Pyramid

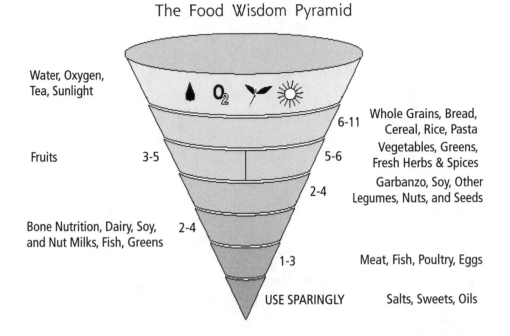

Water, Oxygen, Tea, Sunlight

6-11 — Whole Grains, Bread, Cereal, Rice, Pasta

Fruits — 3-5

5-6 — Vegetables, Greens, Fresh Herbs & Spices

2-4 — Garbanzo, Soy, Other Legumes, Nuts, and Seeds

Bone Nutrition, Dairy, Soy, and Nut Milks, Fish, Greens — 2-4

1-3 — Meat, Fish, Poultry, Eggs

USE SPARINGLY — Salts, Sweets, Oils

ancient cultural wisdom practiced by women around the globe. I have been using this pyramid for over ten years in my work with individuals, health professionals, HMOs, hospitals, and colleges and universities.

OXYGEN, WATER, & SUNLIGHT

The highest level of the pyramid is in the air, because the basis of our life is air, sun, and water. Plants flourish with sun, water, and air and in turn nourish us.

GRAINS

Grains are plant foods that contain starch, soluble and insoluble fiber, protein, antioxidants such as vitamin E and folic acid, and nutrients such as zinc and B_2 that are essential to a woman's health. No wonder whole grains are an important food in most cultures and often are associated with sacred traditions. Many women report that whole grains satisfy their appetites longer than simple carbohydrates like white rice or egg noodles. The sense of fullness comes from the combination of protein and complex carbohydrates that balance insulin and slow down the digestion rate. The glucose released from digesting whole grains enters the bloodstream gradually, giving a pleasant sense of fullness for many hours.

Food Sensitivity to Grains

In my private practice, I have seen hundreds of people show a reaction to grains, particularly wheat. Use of a daily food diary will help you determine if you are sensitive to grains, the specific grains you should avoid, and substitutes you can use instead.

GREENS & VEGETABLES

All vegetables are healthy. Most of them are very low calorie, including culinary herbs, greens, lettuce, celery, and leafy greens. The food wisdom model does not put any limit on the amount of greens, culinary herbs, and other nonstarchy vegetables you can eat. Women need what fruits and vegetables have, and they seldom get enough complex carbohydrates, fiber, phytoestrogens, folic acid, calcium, boron and magnesium, and antioxidants. My multicultural food wisdom pyramid model incorporates all the significant ocean vegetables, a variety of seeds, leafy greens, root vegetables, and color-pigmented vegetables. Many vegetables and greens are rich in vitamins A, C, and E, folate and other B vitamins, and potassium and other minerals. Greens are a super color choice because they are high in calcium and chlorophyll, which is especially good for bone health.

Culinary Herbs & Spices

Culinary herbs and spices stimulate the digestive system, encourage the growth of good bacteria, and affect hormones. Caraway, mint, and licorice, for example, are high in estrogen. Herbs and spices not only make food taste better, but they also have protective antioxidant and phytohormonal compounds with no calories. People should eat as many delicious diverse spices as possible for good health. In some cultures, many herbs, fruits, and even certain flowers are also considered spices.

The low incidence of cardiovascular disease in parts of Spain may be related to the consumption of saffron (Grisolia 1974). Some spices, like cardamom and ginger, can kill up to fifteen different harmful bacterial species (Sherman and Billings 1998).

Every day we are learning more about spices and the many ways they affect hormones and metabolism. Adding spices and herbs in the food pyramid is a new concept, and yet the wisdom for this is age-old.

FRUITS

Although the USDA and other food pyramids list fruits and vegetables together, I believe it is important for you to think of these as separate categories, and to eat many more fruits than usually recommended. Every woman needs at least five servings of fruit and at least seven or more servings of vegetables a day, especially greens and culinary herbs.

BEANS & LEGUMES: LIFE FORCE FOODS

Legumes are at the next level of the pyramid, because they excel in providing the body with the highest quality of soluble and insoluble fiber, plus phytoestrogens. Most people in the world eat grains and legumes more than any other food. Most legumes promote organ and hormone health. They contain phytoestrogens that may help prevent cancer, heart disease, and hormonal fluctuations that can cause PMS and hot flashes associated with menopause. Of all the plant foods, those that are commonly called "beans" contain the most complete and least expensive source of protein. Soybeans and garbanzo beans are about 20 to 22 percent protein, without the cholesterol and fat associated with red meat. Just a cup of cooked soybeans has 18 grams of protein and one cup of garbanzos has 15 grams. An equivalent amount of broiled sirloin has 31 grams of protein, 90 milligrams of cholesterol, and 9 grams of fat. The good news about hearty garbanzos is that they have a low 3 percent fat compared to soy, which yields 40 percent calories from fat.

Nuts & Seeds

Nuts and seeds supply protein and essential fatty acids—the key word is *essential*—for balancing the hormones. A number of the hormones in your body depend on the interaction of fats and carbohydrates.

BONE FOOD

For bone health women need to eat foods that deliver significant levels of boron, magnesium, phytoestrogen, potassium, vitamin D, vitamin K, and zinc because they affect how calcium is used and retained in the body. I looked in many cultures for foods high in calcium, phytonutrients, antioxidants, vitamins, and the minerals needed for calcium absorption, as all of these contribute to healthy bone mass. Dairy foods deliver these, as do many plant foods such as leafy greens and seeds, and nuts. Yogurt is an excellent bone food and good for your health in general.

MEAT, FISH, POULTRY, EGGS

If you enjoy eating meat and eat it often, you can use the following step-by-step approach to substituting plant protein while enjoying the flavor of meat. First, to cut fat choose leaner cuts of meat and eat white poultry meat rather than dark meat. Next, cut the serving amount of meat you eat by one-third whenever possible, by substituting whole grains, legumes, and vegetables as the centerpiece of your meal and positioning the animal protein in the supporting role of the side dish. Then, one day a week use the cleansing way described in chapter 3, and eat no meat.

After you have grown accustomed to eating a third less meat, cut it by another third. Continue substituting and trying new recipes, including soups and stews with small portions of meat. As you observe how you feel, you'll be happy to decrease animal products in your diet. You may always eat meat on special occasions or a few times each week, but you will have substituted other healthy sources of protein, too.

FATS & OILS

The food wisdom pyramid recommends a naturally low-fat way of eating, but some fat is essential to health. Nuts and seeds contain fat, in balance with many other positive elements. It is healthy to use one to three tablespoons of oil in a day, either as cooking oils, in nuts and seeds, or in avocados and olives. Some days you may not use any fat and other days you may prepare a large recipe using two tablespoons of oil but will enjoy it with two other people, or eat it at several meals. I want you to be aware of fats in your diet, but if you are following the food wisdom therapy, you will not have to worry about them.

SUGAR & SALT

If you concentrate on eating whole foods, you will get all the sugar and the salt your body and mind need. Once you adjust to eating according to the food wisdom pyramid, you may never need to flavor with salt or sugar. If you do want to add them, you will use them sparingly. Too much of either becomes a stress to your system. Lack of nutrients signals your body to crave more, leading to a cycle of eating more food without obtaining the elements you need. I call sugar and salt "stressor foods" and urge you to limit them. ❧

balance your health with the pyramid

The food wisdom pyramid helps you bring balance to your body, so you can achieve your best weight, boost your energy, enrich the beauty of your skin and hair, achieve good teeth and bones, strong muscles, and balanced moods, and improve all aspects of your health. By using the food wisdom pyramid, you'll discover what foods you'll want to add to your diet. You'll also discover what foods you might want to eat less of or slowly replace with healthier choices.

After a few weeks of observing how you feel using foods from the pyramid, you'll be able to see that there are changes in the way you feel in connection with the foods you eat. You'll see that healthy choices equal more energy, good sleep, and happier moods. You'll discover that by being attentive to both your body's needs and your own reactions to certain foods you'll prevent problems. Noticing will be the first step toward doing something about it. ❧

the pyramid ways

Food wisdom includes many methods that you will learn to combine on a daily basis.

The planning and food diary way: Finding time each week to look over your food diary, assess your goals, and plan for the week to come is easy when you see how a few minutes will save you time the rest of the week. My kitchen planning tips and recipes can guide you, whether you want to prepare a large celebratory meal or want to eat simple foods without ever cooking—along with everything in between.

The cleansing way: Many cultures enjoy food not only for taste but for cleansing. One day each week, you'll concentrate on using cleansing foods as well as soups and teas to help your body set the stage for healing and nourishing. This cleansing day is a way of using only plant foods for one day to cleanse and rejuvenate based on your individual needs and current dietary practices.

The morning way: Fiber and protein, two crucial components of every diet, are the basis of the breakfast way. If you think breakfast is a bagel or bowl of cereal, wise up! Get ready to experience the variety, color, and flavor of multicultural approaches to this meal. You can have a convenient and nutritious breakfast for weeks without ever repeating the menu.

The tea way: Through my research I have developed a healthful formula for tea that includes a combination of tea, herbs, seeds, spices, and flowers that optimizes energy, stabilizes metabolism, strengthens circulation, hydrates, and cleanses. You'll learn to enjoy tea daily. You'll also learn how to use tea therapeutically and during the seasons to prevent illness and to warm or cool your system. Making your own teas by adding spices, berries, seeds, and herbs as your tastes or needs dictate will seem as natural as choosing your clothes each morning and become an enjoyable part of your daily routine.

The snacking way: Did you ever think a book on food and healthy eating habits would encourage you to snack on and eat as much as you like of some foods? The snacking way is another part of food wisdom that you'll love experimenting with as you incorporate multicultural foods into your diet. Snacks can be seeds, herbs, fruits, grains, vegetables, and spices. You'll be amazed at the variety of flavors and textures that will help balance your metabolism for energy and clarity throughout the day.

The recipe way: This book contains easy, tasty recipes designed to aid your metabolism and to meet your hormonal needs. You will find these recipes balance your system to protect from PMS, hot flashes, insomnia, depression, and other hormonal-related symptoms and help prevent or relieve stress and headaches, build strong bones, aid weight control, and facilitate digestion, respiration, and blood circulation. ❧

the food wisdom model

Chapter 1 introduces hormones, how they interact together and with the various organs and processes in your body to promote good health or to make you ill. You will be encouraged to see your body as a garden, and the food you eat as the nutrients, including air and sunshine that are necessary to make your garden blossom. Food wisdom is about balance and joy in life.

Chapters 2 through 6 give you cleansing and wise eating plans to help you on the food wisdom path. In this section, you'll be encouraged to keep a food diary to help you track your eating habits. You'll also discover how to use new approaches to eating and living that will encourage your body to renew itself, and your mind to rest and rejuvenate.

Chapters 7 and 8 discuss how your specific body processes are affected by foods and how understanding these processes can help you understand your body and any symptoms that may be troubling you. It also presents a therapeutic approach to preventing or relieving common symptoms of hormonal imbalance.

Chapters 9 and 10 include the recipes for foods, snacks, and teas listed in this book, as well as how to use spices to liven up your food, without relying on salt and fat. In this section you'll find old favorites with new flavors as well as new items to try, and you're sure to find recipes you'll love, whether you enjoy spending a day cooking or would rather be anywhere than in the kitchen. ❧

food wisdom goals

To get the most of your own food wisdom program, each week you will be asked to

- *Set three simple goals for the week, based on what you've learned from this book.*

- *Record your food choices and how they made you feel, physically and mentally, in your food diary as described in chapter 2.*

- *Think of change as a great and welcome adventure. If you feel fear or tension, practice breathing and meditation and self-applied acupressure on your body's energy points, as explained in this book.*

- *Cook two food wisdom recipes each month, or one per week, or one each day—your choice.*

- *Celebrate the aromatic, flavorful, colorful, and textured bounty of plant food provided by Mother Earth, sharing the celebration with friends and loved ones, as you connect woman to woman to enjoy one of our basic human needs: food.*

chapter 1

how your hormones work

❧

The body does not have a set time on aging.
We all age if we live long enough, yet some bodies get
old young. Time can be written in our bones.
—Old country wisdom saying

years ago I began to reflect on my own transition to menopause. I wanted to direct my experience to make it as positive a journey
as possible. During my studies for my degree in nutrition, I read so
much about the danger of osteoporosis after menopause that bone health
was foremost on my mind. Osteoporosis, or thinning of bones, is one of
the frequent consequences of menopause as lower estrogen levels result
in reduced protection of calcium in bones. I realized I could be at risk
for osteoporosis because I am lactose intolerant and my mother had
osteoporosis. I also gave birth to my son and daughter as a teenager,
when my own bones were still growing.

My gynecologist wanted to put me on hormone replacement therapy
(HRT) at age forty-two. She thought that certain symptoms I was having might be menopausal symptoms. Like many women, I was reluctant
to begin HRT because it did not seem natural. I did not feel comfortable with the risks associated with HRT, including weight gain and
depression, but particularly the possibility of becoming more vulnerable

to uterine and breast cancer. The role of HRT in women's general health is still being studied.

"If you discover you have good bones, you will need HRT to maintain them. And if you discover you have osteoporosis, you will need HRT to keep the bone you have," my gynecologist reasoned, while telling me I did not need a bone scan.

I asked for a bone density scan anyway, a routine diagnostic test for osteoporosis. Here was another chance to test how eating and exercise had served my body. All my life I had relied on healthy eating and exercise to maintain a sense of well-being. I practiced and benefited from hiking, yoga, qigong, and meditation. When my doctor called to congratulate me on "having the bone density of a thirty-four-year-old," my confidence surged. The food wisdom that I had used and advocated for my clients for two decades was working. I decided to continue with my own eating, qigong, and meditation practices and continued to add to my knowledge of nutrition wisdom from around the world. Before many years passed, doctors were consulting with me about the health and healing benefits of hormonal eating.

Studying the diets of women in other cultures, from country to country, to find out why they did not suffer the same hormonal symptoms as many Western women, I became convinced that changes in the existing food pyramid models needed to be made.

My research, along with my personal experience and observations growing up in several cultures, led me to ask questions. Why are French women usually slim when so many of their recipes are high in cheeses, rich sauces, and carbohydrates? Why do many Chinese women suffer fewer bone problems (such as osteoporosis) even though milk has never been a major part of the Chinese diet? Many Russian women claim to have enormous energy and most Japanese women do not experience weight gain or hot flashes during menopause. What in the Middle Eastern diet keeps women feeling young and vibrant, free of PMS or adverse menopausal symptoms? Do the symptoms and ailments suffered by American women, from starting periods at ever younger ages to weight problems to fatigue to chronic digestion problems to diabetes to osteoporosis, reflect a problem of diet, stress, lifestyle, or exposure to or ingesting of toxins?

American and German researchers reviewing more than two hundred studies concluded that as women's plant food consumption increases, women's risk of breast cancer and all other cancers decrease (Steinmetz and Potter 1996). Plant foods have a similar dramatic effect on heart disease, osteoporosis, and hormone imbalances.

The answer to many of my questions seems to be that, despite what we may imagine is the typical French diet, the French country diet is low in meat and high in vegetables with fruits for dessert. Chinese women build bones with fish and fish bone, tofu, greens, green tea, and other teas. Russian women get energy from yogurt, beef bones, cruciferous and root vegetables, whole wheat grains, and buckwheat. Japanese women use a lot of beans, seafood (including fish bones and seaweed), and green tea. The Middle Eastern diets are high in garbanzos, black tea, greens, yogurt, nuts, and seeds. Commonly in these cultures, meals are vegetable and fruit based, high in fiber, with extensive use of spices and herbs. Meat is used as a condiment. I began to design a food wisdom pyramid and lifestyle for achieving optimal health including oxygen, sunlight, water, teas, spices, and green or culinary herbs, and with an emphasis on diversity. Hormonal eating uses these food choices to keep your hormones balanced. ❧

food & your hormones

Many studies have already established that eating legumes may help prevent cancer, heart disease, osteoporosis, and many symptoms associated with hormonal imbalance.

These studies have proposed that phytohormones known as *isoflavonones*, found in abundance in soy and garbanzo beans, may be one of the principle chemical substances responsible for beneficial hormonal balancing effects. Isoflavones work as enzyme inhibitors and may decrease cancer cell growth in the body. They lower cholesterol levels and have been shown to decrease the risk of heart attacks.

THE NOBLE GARBANZO

Garbanzo beans are rich in protein, nutrients (such as folic acid), fiber, and phytoestrogens. They are a staple food of Middle Eastern cuisine but are not commonly consumed in the United States.

In a 1988 study on the effects of garbanzo consumption on menopausal symptoms, thirty-three American women who were not on HRT were asked to add one cup of cooked, sprouted, and/or roasted garbanzos to their diets for eight weeks. Women reported that the rate and intensity of adverse symptoms of menopause were significantly reduced (70 percent reported a reduction in symptoms by the eighth week). This study appeared to indicate that the addition of garbanzos resulted in a positive health benefit (Gaemi-Hashemi 1988).

Aside from the potential positive effect on menopausal symptoms, garbanzos may have a positive impact on blood cholesterol levels. Blood cholesterol levels also affect estrogen levels. Isoflavones found in garbanzo beans can lower cholesterol by as much as 35 percent (Siddiqui, 1976). Saponins, also found in garbanzos, soy, and other legumes, may lower cholesterol by causing the body to excrete it or by blocking its absorption.

THE MIRACLE OF SOY

How are researchers able to determine the effect of food on hormones? In one example, a test of dietary recommendations for hot flashes looked at the vaginal mucosal cell thickness in women eating two-thirds of a cup of cooked soybeans per day as compared to women who used the estrogen replacement drug Premarin. This test was designed to measure signs of estrogenic activities. The results showed both groups were equally affected. So soybeans can be a preferable alternative to Premarin, which may increase cancer risk, whereas the genistein and other factors in soybeans may lower it (Spicer, Shoupe, and Pike 1991).

Phytochemicals in plants (also known as plant hormones, phytonutrients, or phytohormones) mimic human hormones or evoke a hormonal response, but, depending on the plant source, they have different effects. In November of 2002, *Today's Dietitian Journal* (www.todaysdietitian.com) reported a recent U.S. Department of Agriculture study showing that the culinary herb oregano (one cup fresh) offers forty-two times more antioxidant activity than apples, thirty times more than potatoes, and twelve times more than oranges.

A report on herbs and spices that boost cancer-fighting hormones was given at the 2002 International Research Conference on Food, Nutrition and Cancer in Washington D.C. (Polk 2002). Research on the herb called *angelica* in Europe and *dong quai* in Asian cultures, and which may be found in the United States by both names, shows it has mild estrogenic effects, acts to stabilize blood vessels, and is effective in controlling hot flashes and other menopausal symptoms. Some women experience side effects, so it should be used only on the advice of your own health consultant. ❧

the role of estrogen
& progesterone

Hormonal balance refers to the way estrogen, progesterone, testosterone, insulin, and other hormones entering the blood interact with each other. Hormone production continues after menopause, although menstruation ends, because a weaker form of estrogen, *estrone*, is produced by the adrenal glands. Hormonal balance can be determined by the amount of estrone in the body.

Some estrogen is produced by bacteria in the intestines from foods (such as garbanzos, flaxseeds, beets, lentils, squash, sweet potatoes, and garlic) containing isoflavones and lignans (see discussion later in this chapter). The estrogen *estriol* is produced from estrone in the liver when bacteria in the gastrointestinal tract act on essential fatty acids.

When the hormone insulin is deficient, we may gain weight or become diabetic or depressed. Without progesterone to balance estrogen, some women may develop uterine or breast cancer (Cowen et al. 1981). Too little body fat may result in lowered levels of estrone, and too much body fat storage or production of estrone can make the level too high. Keeping your entire system balanced is certainly a motivating reason for women to maintain a weight healthy for their genetic makeup, body type, bone structure, and lifestyle.

Fluctuations in any one of your hormone levels affect the others and corresponding body functions. The severity of the resulting symptoms can differ greatly from woman to woman.

Progesterone directly affects adrenal and thyroid function, and low levels can result in a drop in blood sugar, headaches, lethargy, depression, water retention, or puffiness.

Estrogen levels tend to drop over time. Menopausal women are often low in estrogen, not because they don't get enough, but because their bodies don't absorb it as efficiently. Premenstrual women have higher levels of estrogen, which can cause PMS symptoms. Most women have experienced bloating or other discomfort before their period or know someone with severe PMS. Certainly almost all women in Western cultures are aware of the symptoms surrounding menopause, including hot flashes, depression, anxiety, distractedness, and insomnia. These are all symptoms of estrogen imbalance.

Many disease and physical discomforts are linked to pre- or post-menopause or PMS, but what many women have not learned is that the foods they eat can be the source of their symptoms. What you eat affects your hormone balance. Garbanzos, black beans, wild yams, tofu, red clover flowers, thyme, licorice powder, or crushed caraway seeds and flaxseeds, among other foods, may help balance your hormones.

Increasing use of phytohormonal foods, such as isoflavonones, genistein, antioxidants, boron, and lignan, to boost the presence of hormones can ease the transition for a woman in perimenopause and during and even after menopause.

Flaxseeds have a hundred times more fiber and phytoestrogens, including lignans, than most other plant foods. Other foods high in phytoestrogens include fennel seeds, celery seeds, parsley, turmeric, and nuts. All can protect you and help reduce adverse hormonal symptoms.⁓

your personal
health concerns

Women are wise to be informed of the illnesses and diseases that can cut our lives short or cause great misery. Your daily habits can have a profound effect on whether or not your body can prevent disease. Think for a minute about your own long-term health goals and the diseases or symptoms that may be a part of your history:

- *Are you concerned about bone density and osteoporosis? Why?*

- *Do you worry that you get enough calcium in your diet? Do you know how to help your body absorb the calcium you eat?*

- *What illnesses are part of your family history? Do you have any specific health concerns, such as breast cancer? Is there a history of cancer in your family?*

- *Do you currently suffer from adverse hormonal symptoms, such as PMS, hot flashes, night sweats, insomnia, anxiety, irritability, digestive and other eating disorders, weight gain, depression, dry skin, or food cravings?*

- *Do you worry about how you will experience perimenopause and menopause? Do you expect to have uncomfortable symptoms or suffer?*

- *Do you want to age gracefully, have vibrant skin, and remain active throughout a long life?*

Again, making wise food choices can improve how you feel. Eating hormonally to balance your systems can be a source of health and symptom healing. ❧

women's need for
balanced hormones

Hormones, secreted into the bloodstream by glands, control the function of distant cells. For example, estrogen regulates our menstrual cycles and influences our sex organs and other vital functions.

Changes in hormone levels make a difference in our sensations, including hunger, moods, and energy. Hormones, these powerful regulators, are especially important to women, as many women in America experience severe, uncomfortable symptoms such as weight extremes, insulin fluctuation, fatigue, and PMS. Research confirms what nutritionists and many women have long believed: physical and emotional symptoms, including bloating, back pain, and mood swings, before and during the menstrual cycle have a physical cause and can thus be treated (Brody 1998).

Studies with my clients have shown that symptoms associated with PMS, uncomfortable menopause, and perimenopause can be alleviated by using a variety of whole phytochemical foods containing fiber. By observing the diets of women in cultures where women have few adverse menopause symptoms, in parts of Africa, South America, and the Middle East, I learned that these women consume legumes, leafy greens, seeds, and yams as a large part of their diets. Further nutritional surveys by other researchers have reported the useful effects of these foods on the hormonal balance in the body, especially during menopause. My Russian grandmother, an expert herbalist in her village, advised women to chew on fennel seeds and cardamom and avoid sugary cookies and candy and coffee to relieve bloating and cramps during their periods. She advised eating herbs, legumes, sprouts, and seeds to alleviate symptoms of hormone imbalance at menstruation and menopause. ❧

hormonal eating is a lifelong process

From the moment our chromosomes determine that we are going to be women, our special nutritional needs begin. Ideally, our bodies are well fed prenatally and in our childhood. In fact, many adult hormonal problems are not the result of aging, but are rather the cumulative effect of years of depriving the hormones of some specific nutritional support they need. Luckily, as I tell my patients, it's never too late to begin! Whatever your current state of hormonal health, eating hormonally can bring you rapid and long-lasting benefits.

HORMONAL FLUCTUATIONS BEGIN EARLY

Hormonal problems can begin as early as our first menstrual period and can lead to such symptoms as migraines, depression, insomnia, mood swings, and fatigue, as well as menstrual problems and fertility issues. Estrogen changes in the menstrual cycle can affect mental performance. Young women do better on verbal memory tests during the luteal phase of their cycle, when estrogen and progesterone levels are high, than during menstruation, when hormone levels are low, as tests by Bruce McEwen (1998) at Rockefeller University have shown. Estrogen increases the number of connections between nerve cells in the hippocampus, a region that is affected by a B complex vitamin, *choline*, which converts to a neurotransmitter. Choline is found in high-cholesterol foods such as eggs and liver (Walis 2003).

We know that what you eat can boost or interfere with mental functioning, enhancing or negatively affecting whatever genetic structure you have inherited. Egg whites, fish (especially cod, dried or fresh), and yogurt are all very good sources of methionine, an essential amino acid that cannot be produced in the body and must be provided by your diet.

JASMINE'S STORY

I first met Jasmine when she introduced herself to me at a conference on women and peace work, where I had been lecturing on the health practices of Russian women. She showed up at my food therapy clinic to combat her symptoms of fatigue, insomnia, mood swings, weight gain, hair loss, aching joints, and dry skin, all of which she attributed to menopause. When she came to me, Jasmine was forty-two and already taking HRT to reduce the severe hot flashes and insomnia she'd been suffering from.

Jasmine kept a food diary for several weeks. As we looked over the records of what she'd eaten, how her energy levels had varied, and how her moods rose and fell, we discovered that she had sensitivities to animal foods, milk, and sugar. We also found that Jasmine's diet was high in animal protein and low in essential fatty acids and antioxidants. She ate almost no seeds, beans, fruit, or spices, and never drank tea. She craved sweets and fatty snacks, and often drank up to five cups of coffee each day.

The first change I asked Jasmine to make was to eat a cup of garbanzos each day in different forms: canned, roasted, and as flour. Jasmine was fortunate in having a husband who loved to cook. Together, the two of them tried recipes with phytohormonal foods, experimenting with yogurt, ethnic spices, and particularly with garbanzos, such as hummus with flaxseed paste and sesame seeds. The flaxseed and sesame seeds provided Jasmine (and her husband) with essential fatty acids, while the phytohormonal foods helped balance her hormones.

After a month or two, Jasmine had become used to adding two or three tablespoons of garbanzo flour and rice bran along with some Asian pear and red berries to her daily Sonia's Antioxidant Smoothie (see chapter 10). So I suggested another change: a daily cup or two of Wise Flower Tea (see chapter 5). Jasmine loved this tea, especially when I told her about some of the cultural traditions on which this formula was based. Jasmine had lived in Moscow for a year and was intrigued by the samovars—large, ornate tea urns—that seemed to be the center of Russian women's lives.

I went on to suggest that Jasmine try a once-a-week cleansing regimen (see chapter 3), eating only green foods one day each week. Although Jasmine would never have considered such an approach when we first started working together, by now she was ready to experiment a little. She said she loved what she described as the light, free feeling she got from cleansing, and she said that the procedure seemed to boost her energy level and improve her mood. She also felt that eating dark green foods fed her sense of "food artistry," inspiring her to experiment with the colors, textures, and flavors of other dishes she prepared.

Finally, I urged Jasmine to learn to meditate. By this point, she was ready for anything, so she took to the practice with enthusiasm. Later she told me that it helped to bring a new sense of serenity and joy into her life.

Over several months, with careful monitoring by her gynecologist, Jasmine significantly reduced her dependence on HRT and eventually stopped using it. Although she reported a few occasional nighttime hot flashes, all of her symptoms had basically disappeared—along with her unwanted weight. In addition, her skin was clear and glowing like never before.

Jasmine continues in good health, with virtually no symptoms and a healthy weight. Even more importantly, she has truly become her own food therapist, listening to her body to learn what choices are right for her. She recently told me, "Although my work has always involved advocating for peace in my community, I've never been at peace with my own body until now."

COLOR CODING FOOD FOR YOUR SYSTEMS' NEEDS

When you look at foods, you can see that they come in an array of vivid colors. Most processed foods have very little brilliant natural color. Sugar, salt, white flour—their plant color is removed in the process. Naturally white foods, such as cauliflower, turnips, parsnips, grapefruit seeds, yogurt, egg whites, white beans, barley, garbanzos, and soybeans nourish your lungs and colon and boost your immune system. The immune system works in conjunction with the hormonal and digestive systems. Try feeding greens to your liver and pancreas to help remove toxins, and eating yellow foods for your spleen and stomach to support your immune system and proper elimination and cleansing.

It turns out that saffron, a vivid yellow spice, may help strengthen the heart (Grisolia 1974). Some high glycemic foods have colors from which you get benefit even though they have a high glycemic index. The yellow beta-carotene in carrots and vitamin C in oranges have been shown to protect us from the effects of low density lipids (LDL), also known as "bad" cholesterol. Recent studies have shown that drinking red wine can have positive effects on the heart, which helps to explain the low incidence of heart disease in the French, although too much wine can also be unhealthy. The flavonoids in red, black, and purple grape skins may be the key. (These studies did not mention that French people eat more fruit and consume fewer calories than many Americans, however, which are both contributing factors.) Food wisdom recommends chewing and eating whole foods—skins and seeds and all—not bioengineered foods or extracts available in capsules. Eat beets, tomatoes, red cabbage, pomegranates, and berries to nourish your heart. Middle Eastern women snack on grapes, seeds, and raisins all day and call them "heaven's food."

Premenopausal women can lower the amount of circulating estrogen by eating foods that provide plant estrogen. Crucifers, for example—a family of vegetables that includes broccoli, green cabbage, red cabbage, kale, brussels sprouts, turnips, purslane, and cauliflower—also contain a variety of antioxidants and are high in fiber, high in beta-carotene, and rich in vitamins A and C, reducing the risk of breast, lung, colon, and uterine cancer. The indoles they contain inhibit the growth of breast tumors (Olsson et al. 1991).

These hardy, brightly colored vegetables withstand poor growing conditions and thrive in cool climates.

LIGNANS

There are two ways for estrogen to circulate through the bloodstream: as free estrogen, which can plug into a receptor site, and as bound estrogen, which cannot. So binding estrogen is one way to keep it from overstimulating our systems. That's what lignans do: they bind with the estrogen circulating in the bloodstream. They also stimulate the liver to produce higher levels of sex hormone-binding globulin (SHBG), which also binds with estrogen. Lignans help balance our estrogen levels in other ways, too. They affect the composition of our intestinal bacteria, which helps to keep our bodies from reabsorbing estrogen. They seem to discourage our bodies from converting fat into estrogen. And studies have shown that a high-lignan, high-fiber, low-fat diet is associated with lower levels of circulating estrogen in premenopausal women (in teenage girls, high levels can manifest as acne), and with a decreased risk of breast cancer (Muti et al. 2000).

Fiber, lignan, boron, and antioxidants perform the crucial task of eliminating estrogens from the bloodstream before they cause damage. A study of perimenopausal women reported the beneficial elimination of estrogen was higher in women eating vegetarian diets, when compared to a corresponding number of women eating both meats and plants (Newcomb et al. 1994).

Women can now test their hormone levels noninvasively with a saliva test kit available from their doctor or pharmacist. Visit www.drsonia.com for more information.

ISOFLAVONES

When diets are high in foods with isoflavones (legumes and vegetables), such as in Europe and the Middle East, the risk of all types of cancer seems to be lower, and these foods' protective effect on hormones may be the reason. Cancer researcher Dr. David Zava made a breakthrough in understanding this process and the hormonal value of eating legumes when he began isolating isoflavones in legumes (Zava, Dollbaum, and Blen 1998). A Greek study showed that women who ate five servings of vegetables each day had a 46 percent lower risk of breast cancer (Katsouyanni et al. 1988). Food choices seem to be the factor in these protective properties, not genetics. Women who move from an area such as China, with low rates of breast cancer, heart disease, and osteoporosis, to an area such as the United States, with relatively high rates, eventually increase their chances of developing breast cancer. Their risk factor increases as they adopt the Western diet. In fact, as Dr. John Glaspy, director of the Bowyer Oncology Center at UCLA, has pointed out, though it's not clear whether diet can prevent breast cancer, we do know that women in industrialized countries have a five times greater risk of breast cancer than women in many Asian countries (Gordon 1998–99).

Isoflavones in legumes resemble estrogen in structure. They can attach themselves to estrogen receptors within the body, acting as surrogate estrogen to balance the fluctuating levels of estrogen released by the sex hormones. Before menopause, these phytoestrogenic compounds become stand-ins for estrogen—like someone taking the place of a high-priced actor to block scenes—and do not require the body to produce as much estrogen. Shorter menstrual cycles and early onset of puberty are connected to the lack of nonsteroidal hormones—the phytohormones in yams, legumes, garbanzos, black beans, and soy—which women in the West do not tend to consume in quantity.

Other phytochemicals such as *genistein*, the main isoflavone found in legumes such as garbanzos, black beans, lentils, and soybeans, have shown numerous antioxidant benefits in preventing disease. Genistein is important in balancing the hormones, can inhibit the growth of tumors, and may even reverse the process that leads to tumors and cancer (Chen et al. 2003). ❧

eating wisely for hormonal balance

Foods that contain high levels of phytohormones and fiber are soy, garbanzos, black currants, beets, flaxseeds, prunes, raisins, lentils, berries, grapes, rose hips, orange blossoms, tofu, grapes, plums, walnuts, cherries, sage, pears, beets, culinary herbs, black beans, buckwheat, peaches, red bell peppers, quinces, kale, spinach, dandelions and other leafy greens, ginseng, red currants, cabbage, tomatoes, and figs. I recommend including three to five of these foods of deep and various colors in your daily menu.

ANTIOXIDANTS, OUR GUARDIANS

Beta-carotene and vitamin C, two powerful antioxidants found in abundance in plant foods, were shown to decrease death rates in a study in Illinois (Pandey et al. 1995). Relative risk of all-cause mortality was 27 percent lower for people who took vitamin C, 20 percent lower for those taking supplements of beta-carotene, and 26 percent lower for combined vitamin C and beta-carotene. The following table of the top thirteen antioxidant foods was adapted from Margen (1992).

Thirteen Powerful Antioxidants

	Vitamin C (mg)	Beta-carotene (mg)	Vitamin E (mg)	Folic acid (mcg)
almonds (¾ cup)	N/A	N/A	21	64
broccoli (1 cup cooked)	100	1.5	2.1	110
cantaloupe (1 cup cubed)	68	3.1	0.3	27
carrot (2 medium)	15	25	0.6	21
kale (1 cup cooked)	60	6.3	8.3	19
mango (1 medium)	57	4.8	2.3	31
orange (1 medium)	70	12	N/A	34
papaya (1 cup)	80	N/A	N/A	49
pumpkin (½ cup)	5	10.5	1.1	15
red bell pepper (½ cup raw)	95	1.7	0.3	8
spinach (½ cup cooked)	9	4.4	2.0	131
sweet potato (1 medium, cooked)	28	14.9	5.5	26

Folic acid may help prevent cervical cancer (Childers et al. 1995). It is found in highest amounts in garbanzos and lentils (one-half cup cooked equals 100 percent of your daily folic acid requirement) and leafy greens, beets, amaranth, and citrus fruits. Since levels of folic acid decrease as we age, older women may need to eat more foods that contain folic acid. One study showed that one three to four ounce glass of wine per day can lower your body's stores of folic acid (Sellers et al. 2001). If you drink, you may wish to add additional greens each day. Folic acid lowers the homocysteine level in the blood, which in turn lowers the risk of cardiovascular disease.

ESSENTIAL FATTY ACIDS: THE VITAL FATS

You can improve your estrogen metabolism by increasing your essential fats. *Essential fatty acids* (EFAs) are specific fatty acids that form part of the cell membranes and are not synthesized by the body; therefore they are "essential" in the diet. Each cell in your body has its own membrane composed of EFAs in the form of phospholipids. The goal of the cell membrane is to keep the cell on an even keel by allowing some hormones and chemicals to flow in through the membrane while other chemicals flow out.

When each cell membrane is working at its peak, each of your cells receives exactly the oxygen and nutrients it needs; responds efficiently to the chemical messages from your nervous system and your endocrine glands; and easily eliminates waste or toxic products. Thus, EFAs increase your hormones and metabolic rate, make your metabolism more efficient, improve the body's ability to use oxygen, and boost energy levels. Over the long term, EFAs can protect against obesity, heart disease, cancer, and autoimmune diseases such as arthritis, AIDS, and many other conditions specific to women during midlife (such as skin, vagina, and hair dryness). People in cultures such as in Japan and Greece, whose diets are high in certain types of fat found in nuts, seeds, olives, and fish oil, have lower rates of cancer of the stomach, colon, prostate, and breast (Tokudome et al. 2000).

By contrast, if you consume large amounts of hydrogenated fats and trans-fatty acids in packaged foods, your membranes become far less fluid. Harmful elements can more easily enter the cell, while beneficial nutrients leak out. Homeostasis becomes more difficult to maintain, and all your cellular processes, including hormonal responses, are disrupted. To make matters worse, these damaged fats tend to crowd out the good ones: they can fit into the same metabolic pathways, but they can't carry out the same biochemical functions. So even if you are taking in some EFAs, their good effects may be blocked by the presence of hydrogenated fats and trans-fatty acids.

BALANCING ESSENTIAL FATTY ACIDS: THE OMEGA FACTOR

Omega-3 fatty acids make hormonelike compounds that may protect from hormonal imbalances such as weight gain, PMS, fatigue, menopausal symptoms, and cancer. Omega-3 fatty acids are found mainly in marine life, although some land plants contain them too, particularly walnuts, flaxseeds, rapeseed (canola oil), wheat germ, and purslane, a green leafy vegetable often eaten in Europe. Very importantly, omega-3s produce substances that break up blood clots, dilate blood vessels, and reduce inflammation, which in turn can help counteract headaches, arthritis, joint pain, and related conditions. Omega-3s may help prevent or counteract the growth of malignant tumors, as well as severe breast-related symptoms in premenstrual syndrome. Omega-6, found in vegetable oil sources (such as corn, safflower, and sunflower oils and animal foods), needs to be brought into interaction with omega-3 to balance it. Omega-3 and omega-6 fatty acids are found primarily in fish, fish oil, nuts (including almonds, peanuts, walnuts, and pistachios), seeds (including flax, pumpkin, sesame, and sunflower), and black currant oil. The U.S. Food and Drug Administration (FDA) validated the claim that one and a half ounces of walnuts a day provides enough healthy omega-3s to boost cardiovascular health and reduce the risk of heart disease (Taylor 2003).

USE FOOD WISDOM TO BALANCE OMEGA-6 & OMEGA-3 FATTY ACIDS

One goal of food wisdom is to balance omega-6 and omega-3 fatty acids in your diet, not least because omega-3 fatty acids can help counteract the inflammatory tendencies of the omega-6 group. Eating flaxseeds and walnuts (an ounce daily) and fatty fish such as salmon, sardines, mackerel, herring, and tuna at least two to three times a week can act directly to create a number of health benefits. Studies show that there may be a correlation between fish consumption and decreases in the incidence of heart attacks (Marckmann 2003). This information underscores the need to get more omega-3 fatty acids in the diet by eating foods that will supply these essential fats. Fish are an excellent source of protein for people who don't want to eat any other animal food. My only concerns about eating fish have to do with the level of toxicity found in so much fish. We need to take serious steps in keeping the earth safe in order to keep ourselves healthy.

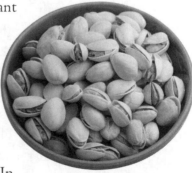

In America we often get too little omega-3 in our diet and too much omega-6, which is found in abundance in animal-based foods. In general, I recommend you consume one to three ounces of omega-3 fat daily through a variety of these foods: sesame seeds, pumpkin seeds, pistachios, peanuts, sunflower seeds, almonds, olive oil, and olives. Eat three to four ounces of fish two to three times a week. I also recommend eating flaxseeds daily. ❧

trans-fatty acids & saturated fat

The most unsafe fats are *trans-fatty acids* or hydrogenated fats, found in foods such as margarine or shortening and in packaged foods such as energy bars, pastries, cookies, and fries. Trans fats may be even worse for you than saturated fats. A simple way to limit trans-fatty acids from our diet is to cut margarine and packaged foods. As awareness of the health risk grows, we must take steps toward labeling. The good news is the FDA is demanding that manufacturers list trans fat next to saturated fat. In Europe, almost all trans fat has been excluded from packaged foods.

Saturated fatty acids are solid at room temperature. Saturated fats come from animal sources (meats and dairy, such as butter) and two vegetable sources (coconut and palm oil). A diet high in saturated fat can result in high blood cholesterol and may result in heart disease. We can reduce saturated fat intake by eating a variety of plant foods and using animal foods only as a condiment. Instead of butter and margarine, try olives, olive or walnut oil, or avocado spread on bread, or nut butters made from almonds, sesame seeds, or walnuts.

One study (Lichtenstein 2003) showed that high intakes of trans-fatty acids might raise blood cholesterol levels, especially LDL cholesterol (the "bad" cholesterol) levels, which affects weight gain. The organ most affected by the kind of fats in our body is the brain. Too much damaged fat such as saturated fat and trans-fatty acid, plus a shortage of EFAs, disrupts the hormonal messages sent by our hypothalamus and pituitary glands, while interfering with our *neurotransmitters*, the biochemicals that transmit messages from the brain to the nervous system. Research has shown that children who are breast-fed have higher

IQs and mood stability then children who are formula-fed, which may be due to EFAs (Gaemi 1992). ❧

food wisdom
for menopause

Women experience menopause differently, just as we are all unique in shape and size and prefer different flavors and colors. Some women report they feel bloated and gassy, and often limiting sugar, starch, coffee, alcohol, and milk (but increasing low-fat organic yogurt and fresh cheese such as unsalted feta, cottage cheese, or ricotta) and adding fiber helps them. Garbanzos, soy, lentils, fruits, vegetables, walnuts, flaxseeds, culinary herbs, and other foods are a good source of lignan and can also help. Some women's good intestinal bacteria may produce more estrogen from essential fatty acids; others have more fat cells that store estrogen, which helps during the menopause stage (Rowland et al. 2000). Some women do take HRT because of their hormone fluctuation; side effects can include headaches, nausea, fluid retention, and increased risk of some types of cancer. ❧

healthy hearts
for women

There is no longer any reason for women to be concerned that they will have heart attacks, high blood pressure, strokes, or blood clotting, problems with risk factors that increase with age. Science has demonstrated that a change in diet can prevent or help heal heart disease, the number one killer of American women (Toobert 2002).

To keep your heart pumping smoothly, your blood flowing, and oxygen fueling all your cells, many nutrients work together—the essential fatty acids of nuts, olives, and grains; the B complex of leafy greens and avocados; the isoflavones of soy and garbanzos; the carotenes of carrots and squash; the folic acid of lentil, garbanzos, strawberries, and boysenberries; the boron of tea and tomatoes; the lignans of flaxseeds, almonds, walnuts, and licorice; the C vitamins in grapefruit; the selenium of mushrooms and seaweed; and the bioflavonoids of beets, pomegranates, and red grapes. The heart delivers oxygen from the lungs to every cell in your body. Your brain, your movements, your digestion, your growth— every one of these activities depends on a fresh supply of oxygen to power it. The vessels and arteries are the body's highways and the flowing blood cells are the suppliers, traveling within the vessels to deliver nutrients and oxygen to all the organs, skin, muscle, and tissue and to transport wastes to be expelled. If fatty deposits left by low-density lipoproteins (LDL), the "bad" cholesterol, clog the highways, the flow of blood decreases. As the deposits grow in size, less blood can flow through, and thus less oxygen is delivered to the cells. The work of the heart becomes more difficult, forcing the same amount of blood through smaller and smaller avenues. The stress of this work can lead to heart attacks.

CHOLESTEROL & FOLIC ACID

Cholesterol is essential for life. It is an important component of cell membranes and is used to manufacture sex hormones, including estrogen and testosterone, and vitamin D (in conjunction with sunlight on our skin). Cholesterol does not dissolve in the bloodstream and must be carried through the blood by proteins.

High-density lipoproteins (HDL), or the "good" cholesterol, transports LDL to the liver to be processed and removed. Most heart disease is caused by LDL cholesterol, which is manufactured in the livers of mammals. Excess amounts can enter our bodies through the animal foods we eat. When estrogen is no longer being manufactured from cholesterol, the amount of cholesterol in the bloodstream increases, and buildups may result. Another contributing factor is the blood level of an amino acid called *homocysteine*.

Folic acid converts homocysteine into less damaging amino acids; vitamins B_{12} and B_6 help with this process. If the conversion does not take place quickly enough because of the absence of these vitamins or a genetic defect, homocysteine can damage arterial walls and promote buildup of cholesterol. For women at risk for heart disease, taking folic acid and choosing foods high in folic acids (lentils and garbanzo beans, for example) will help prevent these problems. A recent Finnish study names iron as perhaps more important than cholesterol, blood pressure, or diabetes as a risk factor for heart disease (Marx 1999). The study found that before menopause women have an extremely low risk of heart disease because they lose iron through their menstrual cycle. After menopause, women start accumulating iron stores in their bodies. Consequently, the heart attack rate becomes similar to that of men. This statistic shows another good reason to limit your intake of meat and poultry, which are high in iron as well as high in cholesterol.

Besides animal food, other factors contributing to the buildup of cholesterol include consuming too many calories overall, taking too many or not enough supplements such as vitamins E, C, and A, and enzymes, not eating enough fiber and phytohormonal foods to cleanse the system, and not getting enough oxygen and exercise to promote a strong heart for circulation. You should not be surprised to find that foods that help prevent PMS or other hormonal symptoms are also good for your heart, and you have learned by now that the presence of protective antioxidants is revealed by the vivid colors of these vegetables.

You can easily address two of the main risk factors leading to heart disease by eliminating (or reducing) animal foods and getting plenty of exercise for your mind and body. If you decrease the amount of LDL cholesterol in your diet, the available HDL will be able to properly dispose of the LDL present. Beginning in the 1960s, a study gathered information about cholesterol levels of middle-aged men in the United States, Greece, and Japan. These same men were watched for twenty years, and the results showed that the Americans, with double the saturated fat intake of the Greeks and five times that of the Japanese, had the highest rates of heart disease and cancer (Tokudome et al. 2000). The Japanese and Greeks had diets high in essential fatty acids and complex carbohydrates, eating more whole grains, beans, and fish. The American Heart Association and the National Cholesterol Education Program suggest eating less animal fat, limiting trans-fatty acids, consuming a variety of fruits, vegetables, nuts, seeds, and whole grains, drinking tea, and doing moderate exercise and breathing exercises to keep your heart healthy and strong. ❧

lowering blood pressure with heart friendly foods

Many of the foods that help to lower cholesterol also have another protective quality: lowering blood pressure. Garlic, celery, carrots, onions, green and black teas, essential fatty acids, fish, nuts, and foods high in vitamin C have all been shown to lower blood pressure, which may prevent strokes (Mayo Clinic 1998). Vitamin C, from oranges, citrus fruits, cantaloupe, chiles, papaya, sweet potatoes, tomatoes, and many other fruits and vegetables, has helped many women lower their risk of stroke. High blood pressure and stroke fatalities are highest among people who eat the least vitamin C. And the more vitamin C, the better.

One study showed that elderly patients who ate one orange a day had twice the risk of high blood pressure as people who ate four oranges.

Potassium foods, such as bananas, potatoes, apples, seafood, adzuki beans, barley, pistachios, plantains, and apricots, can help lower blood pressure and may even lower the amount of medication women with high blood pressure need. In fact, potassium can also help adjust levels of sodium in the body, another factor in maintaining a healthy blood pressure.

High-fiber diets and lots of water, which help eliminate wastes and cleanse the blood, can help lower high blood pressure. Eating the food wisdom way, you will receive most of your sodium from whole plant foods, and so high sodium should not be a concern.

High protein may also encourage your body to store sodium rather than excrete it. If you eat many prepared foods or canned foods and know that there is a history of high blood pressure in your family, you may wish to look for low-sodium alternatives. Nearly 75 percent of the sodium in our diets comes from processed foods. Calcium-rich foods, which help the body eliminate excess sodium, may also help lower blood pressure, and you will already be enjoying those from the bone food tier of the food pyramid. 🍀

foods for strong bones

Osteoporosis, contrary to popular belief, is a disease that can begin in childhood because we need to eat the right foods starting early in life to build and maintain healthy hormones and bone mass in later years. A recent study found that osteoporosis was a major concern of Western women but not a concern in much of the rest of the world (Gaemi-Hashemi 1998). We now know how to prevent bone loss through foods rich in calcium, magnesium, isoflavones, boron, vitamins D, K, B_6, B_{12}, potassium, and phytoestrogens. Many whole plant foods contain both calcium and other components needed for its absorption. To prevent osteoporosis, you should include bone foods and foods with magnesium (tofu, buckwheat, quinoa, rye, parsley, cilantro) and boron (grapes, apple, beets, raisins, nuts, dandelion greens) no matter what else you do to prevent calcium loss.

CALCIUM

The best way for women to absorb calcium is to consume high-calcium foods and foods that increase calcium's absorption. There are also stressor foods that you should avoid because they trigger the release of calcium or block its absorption. Lifestyle risk factors and trigger foods include

- a diet very high in animal protein and refined sugar

- isolated protein (protein derived chemically from foods) such as the soy protein sometimes included in energy bars

- caffeine (one or two caffeinated drinks each day is probably fine unless you are at risk for osteoporosis)

- high-phosphorous foods (which include many canned beverages and sodas, processed cheeses, baked goods, salad dressings, and meat)

- smoking and drinking alcohol

- lack of exercise and meditation

I believe the best way to get calcium into your bones is to encourage the growth of good bacteria in the intestines, and to eat foods that offer calcium in their makeup, especially plant foods: leafy greens and culinary herbs with vitamins K and B, calcium, and boron. A deficiency of vitamin K may cause your bones to lose minerals and can result in bone damage and fractures. Without vitamin K the skeletal structure can be weakened.

Cooked legumes such as garbanzos and soybeans provide as much calcium and protein as milk. A one-half cup serving of spinach, brussels sprouts, and other dark green vegetables significantly lowers the risk of fractures (Feskanich et al. 2002). Sesame seeds, garbanzos, and Sonia's Phytoestrogenic Cereal (see chapter 4) are two other great sources of calcium. Try the hummus recipe (see chapter 6) as well.

Good calcium sources are: broccoli, plain yogurt, garbanzos, milk or buttermilk, soy or almond milk fortified with calcium, kefir (Jewish yogurt), cooked greens (arugula, spinach, kale, or dandelion, collard, mustard, or turnip greens), corn tortillas, sardines, tofu, hummus, cottage cheese, feta, cheddar, Swiss, or Monterey Jack cheese, borani (spinach yogurt), almonds, or sesame seeds.

FOODS THAT AID CALCIUM ABSORPTION

The trace mineral boron reduces the elimination of calcium from the body, helping to keep bones strong. Magnesium, found in abundance in leafy greens, beans, legumes, amaranth, and seeds and nuts, enhances the body's ability to absorb calcium, and the leafy greens and herbs themselves contain calcium. The University of California at San Francisco recently reported that potassium bicarbonate, a compound found in fruits and vegetables such as apples, apricots, beans, seaweed, and potatoes, may help the body retain calcium by neutralizing excess acids created in the body from diets rich in animal foods (Lemann, Pleuss, and Gray 1993). Research continues about the beneficial effects of various plant foods in helping women retain bone mass. Foods that help absorption of calcium for healthy bone are:

Boron: Found in quinces, plums, prunes, leafy greens, strawberries, peaches, cruciferous vegetables (such as cabbage, turnips, and mustard greens), dandelion greens, apples, pears, asparagus, figs, tomatoes, lettuce, berries, cherries, apricots, marjoram, cumin, evening primrose, sage, ginseng, poppy seeds, grapes, beets, tea, wine, and vinegar.

Magnesium: Found in beans and lentils, fugs, spinach, parsley, cilantro, buckwheat, quinoa, potatoes, tofu, wheat germ, collard greens, turnips, nuts and seeds (almonds, peanuts), and milk, yogurt, and other dairy products.

Zinc: Found in amaranth, cashews, almonds, sage, and nettles.

Potassium: Found in potatoes, apples, bananas, beans, Swiss chard, sesame seeds, seaweed, and spinach.

Vitamin K: Found in leafy greens, broccoli, lettuce, spinach, cabbage, oats, green tea, green peas, and brussels sprouts.

Vitamin D: Found in fortified dairy products (including yogurt) and produced by the body when exposed to sunlight.

Vitamin C: Found in black cherries, berries, pomegranates, citrus fruits, tomatoes, garlic, culinary herbs, greens, and tamarind.

I recommend that my patients take enzyme supplements to encourage the growth of healthy bacteria in the intestines, which helps the body absorb calcium efficiently. ❧

integrating east & west for body, mind, & spirit

A restorative approach to healthy hormones includes eating mindfully, eating foods that are a treat to our senses, cleansing, building healthy stores of good bacteria, and balancing and treating specific problems of the body through food and nutrition. When I was a child, the women in our town recommended white vegetables for a sore throat, earache, or infection in the digestive tract. Even as a child, I could see that these foods helped. Later, through research, I understood how starting the day with white pears (including chewing and eating the seeds), having a lunch of barley soup (including turnips and mushrooms), and finishing the day with cloves of garlic helped to get rid of infection, inflammation, or digestion problems. Tea, garlic, and garlic-family foods have antibacterial properties and contain the phytonutrient *allicia*; cabbage and cauliflower contain phytonutrient *indoles* that regulate hormones and prevent disease. Turnips, licorice root, lily bulb, pear skin, ginseng, red yeast rice, and tumeric are highly prized as anti-inflammatory agents. Both Chinese and Middle Eastern traditions connect the healing qualities of all these foods with certain symptoms, but they use different methods to describe them. The way they choose to identify the foods, either by color or heat properties, is a shorthand for understanding the desired effect of each food. Science has now shown that these vegetables help to cleanse the body and restore the proper balance of bacteria in the digestive tract, so the body's own bacteria-fighting agents can take over and rid the system of the underlying infection.

Another aspect of Eastern thought that is being incorporated into Western medicine is the connection of the body, mind, and spirit. Too often, women treat symptoms such as PMS with pills that ease pain or reduce bloating without looking at the stress in their lives or lack of nutrients in their diets that may exacerbate or contribute to physical discomfort. The food wisdom approach asks you to examine all the possible underlying causes, including hormonal imbalance caused by diet, stress that affects your adrenal glands and robs your body of vitamins and nutrients, or too much caffeine or sugar that causes imbalances in blood sugar and hormones. As you think about your own food and health practices, connect your entire being: your senses, your emotions, your tastes, your desires, your thoughts, and your goals. Balance your physical, emotional, spiritual, and intellectual self with your environment, the foods you eat, your home, family, friends, work, the weather, the times in which you live, and the larger world of nature surrounding it all.

chapter 2

food wisdom for life

We who are luminous, are radiant, are 90 percent light,
who know a fiery fusion that makes stars and suns,
whose flesh is compressed of dancing atoms.
—Mary Rudge

food choices and decisions sometimes seem a burden to many women, and often we eat based on convenience, rarely evaluating the true benefits of meal planning and wise eating. Many of us do not spend time planning foods for ourselves and our family, or observing how we feel when we eat certain foods. But a wise shopping plan can make healthful tea, breakfast, and snacking as convenient as any foods you now use. Planning and eating mindfully are easy, with color, flavor, and a little shopping to set the stage. Food planning helps you economize time and money by focusing on the value of choices for your health.

By selecting and mastering three to five basic recipes from this book, planning meals will be easier. Consciously choosing two or three colors for every meal will change your attitude. Soon, adding green, red, yellow, brown, orange, and other colors of foods will come naturally. The more you use food wisdom, the more confident you will be and the better you will feel. ❧

making the kitchen the center of busy lives

Today's hectic lifestyles have made the kitchen as a gathering place all but obsolete, but we can use the conveniences we have in the modern era to reestablish the kitchen as a nourishing environment. We no longer assume that a woman's only job is to keep the family well, but wellness for all is still a primary goal of loving care, and we can re-create some of the sacred, joyous aspects of the traditional kitchen in our own homes.

It takes only a few minutes each day to plan ahead and to look back at the foods you have eaten and the way you felt afterward. These few minutes can actually save time in the end, as you prepare shopping lists and think about a recipe that may provide meals and leftovers—what I call *encore meals*.

In this chapter, you will learn ways to save time while incorporating healthier habits into your diet. If you follow even a few of these suggestions, I promise that you will find joy in your own kitchen, and that joy will spill over into meals shared with friends and family. This chapter is designed to help you set up your kitchen for food wisdom ways in only a few minutes a day. ❧

keeping a food diary

Few women would dare leave the house before checking their hair, makeup, and clothing in a mirror. Even the least vain of us share a need to verify what we've put on our bodies before we meet the world. Unfortunately, not as many of us spend that same few minutes reflecting on what we put *into* our bodies each day. Begin your path to food wisdom with a single, simple step. Today, begin a food diary.

Keeping a food diary provides you with reflection time and serves as an interior mirror showing how the type of food you eat and beverages you drink make you feel—mentally and physically—over the course of your day. Your food diary serves you three ways. It helps you discover the most pleasurable aspects of food for you. It helps you see how the foods you eat and beverages you drink may be causing you harm. Finally, continued use and review of your food diary helps you realize the habits that are not serving your long-term physical needs and replace them with wiser and healthier choices.

HOW TO BEGIN

Start with a simple approach of writing down each item you eat over the course of one week. Once you establish the writing habit, you'll find it a process that takes just a minute or two after each meal and snack. The benefits of doing this will far outweigh the price of a few moments of your time.

WHAT TO LIST

Throughout the day list each item you consume. As much as possible, record the portion of each item. Rather than just writing that you drank coffee, it is better to write "8 ounces of coffee with ¼ cup half-and-half." The same is true with food. If you have a lunch salad, write "large bowl of mixed greens, tomato and cucumber slices, the juice of one fresh lemon, 1 tablespoon blue cheese dressing mixed with ¼ cup yogurt." The more details you include, the more you will learn from this practice. If you cook from recipes, you can simply note the name of the dish. If you later need to track the specific ingredients, you can verify them from the recipe. When eating in a restaurant, try as much as possible to note what you had, any unusual ingredients in the dishes, and the approximate portions you enjoyed.

WHERE YOU EAT IS IMPORTANT

Where and how you eat also impact how you process your food. If you think, "Orange juice just doesn't agree with me" or "I don't like orange juice," for example, consider where and how you drink orange juice. Gulping some questionably fresh orange juice from concentrate straight out of the container while standing in front of the refrigerator is a very different experience than sipping fresh-squeezed organic orange juice from a goblet while you watch the birds fluttering in your backyard. It's the same food item in the food diary, but a world of difference in how it is consumed.

WHEN YOU EAT CAN MAKE A DIFFERENCE

Make a quick indication of the hour and minute you ate or drank each item. It is much better to note the exact time rather than simply indicate breakfast, lunch, or dinner. Timing is especially important if you are trying to track the cause of a problem that you think may be food related. Between-meal snacking can be a source of problems for many women attempting to control their weight. While their meals are sensible, their snacks become obsessive. You may find from writing down the time you snack in your food diary that the timing of your meals should be adjusted. Perhaps because you eat breakfast at seven in the morning, it is really time for lunch by eleven thirty and not time for a sweet indulgence. Eating late at night may cause indigestion that hinders sleep for many people. If you have insomnia, noting the time of your evening meal and later comparing it to how you sleep could indicate a dining schedule change is all that is necessary.

WRITE DOWN YOUR LEVEL OF ENJOYMENT

Indicate the level of enjoyment you gained from the meal or snack, using a numbered scale. Thinking of the finest, most enjoyable meal you've ever had as a 10, and the worst meal as a 1, and indicate in your diary the rating for each item you consume. Over time, you can track the eating style that you really don't enjoy and strive to eliminate that method from your life. Giving a meal a high rating doesn't necessarily mean that the meal was shared with Mr. Right in an expensive restaurant, or that the snack was something outrageous eaten on the beach at sunset: it is whether or not you enjoyed the meal at the time.

FOLLOW YOUR REACTIONS

Check into your diary again about an hour after you eat or drink. Stop for just a minute and see how you feel. Next to the last entry, indicate both your general mood and your short-term physical condition. Are you sleepy or energized? Cranky or happy? Nauseous, bloated, or content? Do you have a headache or sinus trouble? Do your joints hurt or is your stomach upset? Are you feeling patient and understanding with coworkers and kids or are you ready to give the world a time-out? Your reactions may relate back to both what you ate and the enjoyment of the meal.

Food sensitivities often come on quickly. If you regularly react unpleasantly after eating the same food, you can cut it out of your diet for a while to see if this clears your problem.

By tracking your physical and emotional feelings every few hours in your food diary, you can get a handle on the food and beverages, mealtime, and eating style that work for you and those that cause you problems. 🏵

recording methods

There are no right or wrong ways to make your food diary. The food diary I use contains space to write down all of the elements detailed above: *what* I ate or drank, *how much* I consumed, *where* I ate, *when* it was consumed, my *enjoyment rating*, and my later *reaction* and *energy level*. You can rate your energy level and the intensity of the symptoms you are having from 1 to 10 with 10 being the highest intensity of the symptoms you feel. Using the same sheet, I record my *daily exercise* type and amount, the quality and amount of *water* I consume and quality *air* I breathe, the quality and quantity of *sleep* I got that night, and my *general thoughts and feelings* of the day. 🏵

you can diagnose problems

Once you have established your food diary, use it to diagnose your biggest problems first. Compare your physical symptoms and emotional feelings on days when you have made wise food choices against those on days when you have let unhealthy temptations rule your decisions. See how your eating habits—what, where, when, and with whom you eat—affect how your body uses the food and drink you consume. Also check the influence of individual foods and beverages on your immediate health and personality.

College sophomore Sabrina suffered from stomach pains followed by diarrhea regularly. Her campus health center told her it was stress and recommended a prescription drug to elevate her mood. Although she had a lot going on in her life at the time, including a full school schedule, a part-time job, friends, roommates, and a boyfriend, she didn't feel particularly stressed. Her dance classes and good relationships kept her life in pretty good balance. She was reluctant to take a drug to solve a problem and frankly couldn't afford the regular cost of the prescription. Instead, she chose to track when the stomach problems occurred. Adding a food diary to the journal she was already keeping for an English class, she noted what and when she ate, and also noted when the stomach problems occurred. When she looked through her diary she found that the stomach upset occurred three times the first week: after a morning muffin with hot chocolate, after sharing a banana split on a movie date (really ruining the romantic mood of the evening!), and after a smoothie sipped one day in class. Because all these entries contained dairy, she thought perhaps she was lactose intolerant, cut out all milk products for a week, and continued keeping her food diary. Unfortunately, the stomach problems continued this week after eating some nut bread her roommate baked and after a nondairy smoothie. Reviewing the ingredients that were consistent in both weeks, she realized that the pains always began about an hour after she ate banana, which the campus added to all its smoothies and which her roommate and the cafeteria had used in baking. Once she eliminated bananas from her diet, the stomach problems disappeared. While bananas are generally a healthy item, for people like

Sabrina, an intolerance for them can be problematic. Keeping a food diary for just two weeks saved her countless days of pain.

DR. SONIA'S FOOD DIARY ENTRY

Today is a gift: I meditated 5 minutes in thanks.

A glass of Sofia's Seeds and two glasses of water. Played tennis for 35 minutes with 5 minutes standing meditation and 10 minutes weight lifting.

Breakfast:

multigrain rye bread	1 slice
feta cheese	1 oz.
fresh basil	2 cups or 1 bunch
almonds and pecans	few ~ 10 each
Asian pear	1 med.
Healthy and Wise Tea	4 cups

Level of enjoyment: 8

Snack:

deep breathing	5 minutes
watermelon	1 slice
roasted flaxseeds	2 pinches
chai latte with soymilk	1 cup

Level of enjoyment: 7

Lunch:

Fish steamed with dandelion greens	1 slice (2 oz.)
and black beans	1 cup
Sonia's Phytoestrogenic Cereal	1 cup
fresh peach with yogurt	1 med. and ½ cup

Level of enjoyment: 8

Snack:

deep breathing	5 minutes
Tea for Life	1 cup
garbanzos (roasted)	¼ cup
cookie shared with friend	2 small bits

Level of enjoyment: 7

Dinner:

baked beets	1 med.
sweet potato	1 small
French bread	1 slice
buttermilk with dried mint	½ cup

Level of enjoyment: 9

Snack:

daily journal writing	5 minutes
soybeans (steamed)	½ cup

Level of enjoyment: 8

As you can see, I got my protein from yogurt, nuts, legumes, grains and nuts and seeds. I got plenty of fiber and isoflavones from my tea, legumes, cereals, and herbs. I got enough spices in my tea and by adding extra anise, cumin, fennel, and cardamom to my yogurt, salad, cereal and tea. The beans I used were marinated (sometimes I choose roasted, baked, or another style of preparing). What I am missing or not getting adequately are greens, even though I've had some dandelion greens, mint, and basil. I'll keep this in mind as I plan for more greens in tomorrow's meals. ❧

realize your food wisdom goals

Continue to review your food diary regularly to track your progress along the path. Do not let a day or even a week of forgetting to write stop you from continuing your diary. As you read this book, I want you to incorporate centuries of food wisdom into your daily life. You can't expect to make changes overnight or fail to slip into old habits occasionally. Just stay open to learning the food wisdom ways and you will do well.

SHARING YOUR INFORMATION

Your diary is a private document that you create to bring wisdom into your world. That said, you may want to share your knowledge with others. If a health symptom continues despite changes in your eating habits, you should consult a physician, bringing your food diary with you. Any dietitian, nutritionist, or other health care provider will gain a great deal of knowledge about you from reviewing your eating habits over time.

CREATING YOUR OWN FOOD HAVEN

You have been paying attention to your food diary and learning much about the type and quantity of foods you eat. But have you given much thought to the way in which you prepare and eat foods, or how to plan ahead to have all the right foods conveniently at hand? Take a minute to answer the following questions:

- *Do you plan for the week before shopping, or simply buy whatever catches your fancy?*

- *Do you enjoy your kitchen and take time to make it pleasant? If not, what are the reasons?*

- *How much time do you spend in food preparation or in the kitchen each week?*

- *What foods are displayed in your kitchen for easy access? What is in your refrigerator? What utensils or objects are displayed?*

- *Do you plan shopping for teas and snacks, preparing to have ingredients on hand?*

- *Do you have whole grains, rice, dried legumes, and other food wisdom foods ready to use in soups and stews, for breakfast, and for quick meals?*

- *How often each week do you go to the cupboards and find no healthy foods to eat?*

- *Would you like to share meals with family and friends more than you have a chance to do?*

- *Do you eat alone often? Do you sit down and enjoy your food, or do you eat quickly, reading or watching television and rushing off to the next task?* ❧

your kitchen: the heart of your home

As with many human endeavors, creating balance and harmony takes planning, skill, and patience. Just as certain foods can bring balance and harmony to your body and mind, certain practices and techniques can bring ease and joy into your kitchen. Even simple planning, like having healthy bunches of fresh herbs on hand for nibbling or drying will make a difference in your life. My friend Katherine visited my home, and I immediately made her a tea with a pinch of fresh herbs and spices from my "condiment tray." I quickly warmed roasted root vegetables—deep purple beets, bright orange sweet potatoes, and creamy white turnips—in the oven. I served these on a plate beside leaves of arugula, tarragon, and green onions, added yogurt on the side, and sprinkled the veggies with a mixture of flaxseeds and sesame seeds. In moments, we had lunch, and Katherine said, "I wish I had this type of loving lifestyle to keep me healthy and at peace."

I told her how easy it was: it is just as easy to buy fresh greens and herbs as packaged foods. We made a shopping list for her and she took the recipe for roasting root vegetables and enjoyed it later.

Not every woman will adopt each of the user-friendly suggestions offered here; you may adopt some ideas and discard them later as you develop your own techniques and preferences. Please accept these suggestions as you would a cup of tea in my kitchen, with an open heart, an open mind, and a loving, willing attitude.

SETTING EATING PRIORITIES & SHOPPING PATTERNS

Your goal for the kitchen should be order, convenience, and calm enjoyment. Have you ever entered a kitchen that welcomed you and made

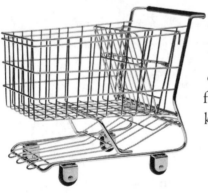

you want to begin preparing food? Those kitchens have fresh ingredients openly displayed and gleaming utensils at hand. In my kitchen, I keep a ceramic vase with a bouquet of fresh culinary herbs on the countertop. The fragrance greets me each time I walk into the kitchen and inspires me to nibble on greens.

Kitchens around the world are full of jars of spices and bowls of fruit. When they first see my long food shopping lists, some women tell me that they have no room to store all these foods. They soon discover, however, that fresh fruit in a basket replaces the cookies in the cupboard, and that rice and a few greens are as convenient as frozen dinners. They no longer need room for six-packs of canned sodas in the fridge. Their freezers fill up with cooked grains and encore meals, and their refrigerators contain fruit and tea ingredients.

Choice and planning can change your kitchen and menu planning, too. Keep the foods you want to eat in front of your eyes and in easy reach and keep the tools you need at hand. Without these, cooking will never be fun and the nourishment you receive will be negated by the stress caused by preparing it.

SETTING SMALL GOALS: TINA'S STORY

Elizabeth, a successful broadcast journalist in the Bay Area, was one of those women who had never felt comfortable in the kitchen or learned basic cooking skills. She ate most of her meals in restaurants. In addition, Elizabeth suffered from irritable bowel syndrome (IBS).

Elizabeth started making bacteria-friendly tea and eating fruit in the morning and trying one simple recipe each week. She stopped at restaurants and bought soup, brought it home, and ate it with a fresh sauté of vegetables and tofu. Week by week, her IBS improved and she cut down on her medication.

Elizabeth eventually realized that one of the reasons she liked eating in restaurants was that she was lonely. She solved this problem by inviting two friends to join her on Sunday for a day of experimenting with eastern Mediterranean recipes. Now, every few weeks the women meet at the local farmers' market on Sunday morning, shop for ingredients, and go back to one woman's apartment to cook, talk, and have fun. At the end of the day, they have indulged themselves in amusing and meaningful conversation, jokes, laughter, and mutual support. They practice qigong, yoga, and meditation together, play music and sing, and all have healthful foods to take home for the week.

A MASTER SHOPPING LIST FOR THE WISE WOMAN EATING WITH JOY

Shopping and storing foods are crucial to keeping your life easy and your cooking spontaneous yet creative. If you don't have the basics, you will have trouble preparing any meal. If your supplies go bad before you use them, you will be frustrated by wastefulness, and you may find yourself stuck in the middle of a recipe. Here are a few suggestions to get you started with the basics of shopping and storing:

- For each week, concentrate on a few different types of foods and combinations of these foods.

- To vary the taste of your meals, add new spices and condiments.

- To add variety, add different side dishes such as fruits, vegetables, cheese, or yogurt.

- Pick out a food such as garbanzo beans, and try to see how many different ways you can eat them.

- Use the shopping list included at the end of this chapter to guide your shopping selections.

- Plan your meals ahead of time, so you don't buy foods that are unnecessary.

THE ADVENTURE OF MULTICULTURAL SHOPPING

To make shopping as much fun as possible, I often travel to different areas of town and explore. I now have a favorite tofu, seaweed, and mushroom store. At Chinese and Vietnamese markets, I listen to music and language, observing what people put into their baskets and their attitude toward food. My shopping day is a day I experience multiculturalism, connecting to people and taking care of myself by expanding my choices. Think of incorporating this multicultural experience into your life as a food adventure journey.

The monthly shopping list at the end of this chapter is comprehensive. You may want to begin by buying three or four things from each section each week until you build up your supplies. Pick a few recipes, and make sure to buy everything you need for them; then add a few more ingredients to expand your choices. Use the list each month to take stock and to restock.

You might want to make the first month "Italian month" by buying mostly herbs and pastas used in Italian cuisine, and then move on to other ethnic and cultural choices.

- Italian cuisine: anise, basil, crushed red pepper, fennel, garlic, oregano, rosemary, sage, pasta

- Chinese cuisine: ginger, sesame seeds, white pepper, whole red chiles, garlic, crushed red pepper, curry powder

- Thai cuisine: basil, cilantro, cinnamon, mint, turmeric, lemongrass

- Greek: cinnamon, dill, mint, onion, oregano, paprika, olives

- African: yams, lentils, bananas, dates, couscous, injera bread

- Persian/Afghan: cumin, cardamom, turmeric, garlic, tarragon, licorice, fenugreek, fennel, flaxseeds, saffron, garbanzos, tahini, black sesame seeds, yogurt, raisins

- Japanese: miso, seaweed, soybeans, tofu, eggplant, citrus

- Mexican: cayenne pepper, cilantro, cinnamon, cumin, jalapeño peppers, black beans, tortillas

- Indian: curry powder, lentils, fruit chutney, white radishes, cloves, nutmeg, cumin seeds, mustard seeds

Do buy fresh herbs and greens as much as possible. These are available year-round: parsley, dill, peppermint, seaweed, mint, spinach, bok choy, cabbage, all types of lettuce, kale.

Although you may think that buying fresh or organic foods is more expensive than your usual way of shopping, over time you will see that the food value far exceeds the monetary value. Fresh nuts may seem expensive, but are usually less per pound than meat and go much further. Some clients use small-farm delivery services to have fresh, organic vegetables delivered to their door each week. Many of these services provide recipes for preparing unusual vegetables, such as purslane or rutabaga, and might be a good option if you haven't used fresh vegetables often. Explore ethnic markets and use their delis to learn about new foods and new ingredients. Over time, you'll incorporate more and more foods from the list, and each new addition will be easy.

READING LABELS FOR YOUR PEACE OF MIND

Although I recommend that you buy most of your foods whole, and preferably organic, you will be purchasing some prepared foods. Recently, the FDA revised the requirements for ingredient and nutritional labeling on foods with the intent of helping consumers make informed decisions. Unfortunately, some of the changes have added confusion. For instance, the daily value (DV) of nutrients assumes an intake of 2,000 calories and the percentages are what percentage that food will provide of your DV of a specific nutrient (such as fat) that day, not the percentage of that nutrient in the food. For example, a carton of sour cream labeled as "light" with a 3 percent DV of fat is actually 57 percent fat calories, but one serving amounts to 3 percent of the FDA recommended 65 grams of fat per day. You should be attentive to the number of servings per container, too, and the serving size. Here are a few terms that have been clearly defined by the FDA and what they mean on labels:

- High-protein: must contain at least 10 grams of protein per serving.

- Good source of calcium: contains at least 100 milligrams of calcium per serving—almond or soy milk contains 30 percent of the daily value for calcium and more than 5 grams of protein.

- Sugar-free: less than 0.5 grams of sugar per serving.

- Light for fat means 50 percent less fat than a comparable product.

- Light for calories means 33 percent less than comparable product *and* 50 percent less fat.

- Light for sodium means 50 percent less than a comparable product.

- Low-fat: no more than 3 grams of fat per serving.

- Low-calorie: 40 calories or fewer per serving.

- Low-sodium: 140 milligrams or fewer per serving.

- Good source of a nutrient means it contains 10 to 19 percent of the RDA for that nutrient.

Vitamins and supplements should include a USP label, which means it meets the standards of the U.S. Pharmacopeia testing organization (although they cannot really measure absorbability of the vitamins). Look for the following:

- cereals with at least 3 grams of fiber per serving (many brands contain 10 or more grams, helping you meet the recommended 35 to 45 grams per day)

- active bacteria in yogurt (if packages bear the National Yogurt Association's label reading "live and active cultures," the yogurt must contain ten million live organisms per gram)

There are certain types of sugars, fats, and additives that you should avoid if possible:

- trans-fatty acids or hydrogenated fat

- aspartame

- olestra

- artificial colors, sweeteners, or flavors

In general, using food therapy's principles makes life easy when you buy whole colorful foods and eat them whole or prepared with a small amount of olive oil, salt, sugar, spices, herbs, and vinegar. As long as you are eating healthy, it is okay to buy some prepared foods. However, try to buy them in small portions.

Beware of the advertising gimmicks that some food manufacturers use. Be careful of low-fat, light, nonfat, sugarless, decaffeinated or diet foods, because they involve too much processing. Usually low-fat or nonfat desserts mean lots of sugar or artificial sweeteners and fats. Food wisdom encourages you to minimize processed sugars and fats.

ENCORE FOODS FOR BUSY WOMEN

Encore foods are recipes prepared for more than one meal at a time. Just like an audience may demand more from a wonderful performer until another piece is offered, encore foods are foods so good you want to eat them another day. Many of my food wisdom recipes include left-overs for freezing. I recommend you use one or two hours every few weeks to prepare a recipe, doubling it if desired, and freeze the remainder to be used for meals and take-along lunches later in the week or month. Cooked legumes freeze particularly well.

If you are preparing a meal with pasta, freeze only the sauce and make the pasta fresh at the time you prepare the encore meal. For a red sauce, you can sprinkle herbs, feta cheese, and diced tomatoes on top.

FOOD WISDOM SUBSTITUTES

Here are a few ideas for healthy shopping and eating alternatives:

- Buy plain active-culture yogurt and use as you might use sour cream.

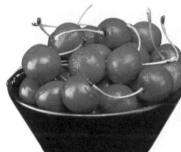

- Buy fresh fruits instead of sweets.

- Add tofu or beans to stews instead of meat, or cut meat by half.

- Make a root vegetable kabob to grill in the summer instead of meat kabobs.

- Buy fruit jams to use on toast rather than butter.

- Buy fresh carrots to munch instead of chips.

- Use powdered or chopped licorice root to sweeten tea rather than sugar.

- Buy brown rice to use instead of white bread to accompany meals.

Frequent restaurant patrons eat 25 percent fewer fruits and vegetables. How about starting a new trend, a trend toward eating more fruits and vegetables in restaurants? Create your own "take-along" encore meals with healthy snacks and portable breakfast choices, and use these foods to supplement or take the place of purchased foods. Whether you are planning to eat in restaurants, going on a picnic or to a party, or preparing a brown-bag lunch, the following tips can help you eat well anywhere you go:

- Prepare your lunch when you fix dinner by putting a portion in a take-along container to reheat at work.

- Prepare a month's worth of travel snacks to keep at your desk.

- Sardines, roasted root vegetables, beans, cucumbers, berries, hard-boiled eggs, fresh fruits, yogurt, whole wheat bagels, and carrot sticks make great picnic fare.

- If you are going to a party or restaurant, think about what you will eat before you go and eat an appetizer of fresh colorful fruit or culinary herbs beforehand to balance other choices; this is especially useful if you are hoping to eat less of too-rich or calorie-laden party foods.

- If you are going to a potluck party, prepare a lentil salad, a plate of raw veggies, or a fruit salad. Your friends will appreciate it.

- When you travel, take along nuts, roasted garbanzos, and dried fruit to snack on.

DIET FOR JET LAG

If you are traveling through different time zones, use food to help you stay alert and sleep well at night. The day and evening before, eat plenty of complex carbohydrates—fruits, vegetables, and grains. The morning you leave, drink Sophia's Seeds Formula, (see chapter 3) eat fruit, and carry more seeds and fruit to nibble in transit. Once there, rest as much as possible and then eat protein to get moving again. If you feel run-down, use Sophia's Seeds Formula to cleanse your system. ❧

food wisdom
planning goals

Take a moment to set goals for the following week based on what you have learned in this chapter. Here are a few sample goals to get you started:

- *"This week I will make a shopping list and buy fresh grains to use for breakfast."*

- *"This week I will buy five types of fruit to use in smoothies and experiment with different combinations."*

- *"One weekend this month, I will prepare a new food wisdom garbanzo pilaf, and freeze half for the next week."*

- *"I will invite a friend to go shopping with me for legumes and rice and explain the phytohormonal benefits of plant protein to her."* ❧

a wise shopping list

Use this list when you go grocery shopping. Buy as many of these items as you wish. Try to buy at least two to three items from each section each time you buy groceries.

Dried fruits: apricots, assorted berries, bananas, dates, figs, pears, peaches, plums, prunes, raisins (choose fruits in a variety of colors)

Legumes: white beans, baby and long limas, black-eyed peas, garbanzo beans, kidney beans, lentils, mung beans, navy beans, split peas, bean sprouts

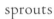

Beverages: mineral water (sodium-free), club soda (sodium-free), spring-water, buttermilk (low-fat), tomato juice, pomegranate juice

Oils: olive and virgin olive oil, vegetable, peanut, safflower, walnut, roasted sesame, almond, pistachio, grape seed

Herbs and spices (dried): anise seeds, basil, bay leaves, cardamom (ground), cayenne pepper, celery seed, chili powder, chives, cinnamon stick and powder, seaweed, tarragon, sage, turmeric powder, thyme, saffron, sumac, rosemary, paprika, pepper, coriander seeds or powder, cumin, dill seeds, fennel seeds, fenugreek, garlic, ginger, lemon peel (dried), lemon balm, chopped licorice root, mustard, oregano, peppermint, caraway seeds

Grains and starches: amaranth, quinoa, bulgur, barley, buckwheat (roasted), cornmeal, couscous, spelt, millet, red potatoes, cornstarch, whole wheat flour, lasagna noodles, pasta (spaghetti and other noodles), bread crumbs, soy milk powder, jasmine rice, wild rice, brown rice, roasted garbanzos, all-purpose flour, corn flour, soy bran, barley flakes, rice bran

Nuts: almonds, chestnuts, peanuts, pine nuts, pecans, pistachios, walnuts, peanuts, hazelnuts

Seeds: flaxseeds, pumpkin seeds, poppy seeds, sunflower seeds, tahini, sesame seeds, black sesame seeds

Dry or sprouted seeds: khak shir seeds, basil seeds, psyllium seeds, red clover seeds, fenugreek seeds, alfalfa seeds

Tea: green, black, red (rooibos), white, herbal, borage

Canned and other foods: beets, tuna, sardines (water-packed), lemon juice or lime juice, pickles (in vinegar, low-salt), tomato paste or sauce, wine, miso, natural licorice or ginger candy, pineapple chunks, ketchup, horseradish, applesauce (unsweetened), relish, salsa, mustard, rice cakes, tomatoes (whole, canned, or dried), healthy vegetable or bean soups, vinegar (rice, seasoned, balsamic, wine, fruit, or herb-flavored), and garbanzo, soy, kidney, black, and other beans

chapter 3

the cleansing way for energy & health

*The cell is immortal! The cell does not deteriorate nor grow old
if the elimination of wastes and proper nutrients are maintained.*
—Alexis Carrel, Nobel Prize winner

renewal takes place within, even if we do not see it. Cells grow, do their work, and are replaced. Foods are digested and broken down into useful chemicals or waste and moved through the body accordingly. Energy is created and wastes excreted. Unused fluid and food residue can move through the skin, colon, and urinary tract. Your immune system and digestive system must slough off old cells, unneeded vitamins and extra iron, and other unneeded or harmful substances.

Cleansing helps protect your system from environmental toxins. Eliminating accumulated food waste through a cleansing day will allow your digestion to better utilize the fiber, antioxidants, phytohormones, and other nutrients from foods to recharge your immune system, your hormones, and your metabolism to promote health. Eating well keeps you feeling young and helps prevent many illnesses.

The first step to optimum health and high energy is to strengthen your body by assisting the digestive, urinary, and respiratory systems in eliminating wastes. Next, you must help maintain healthy enzymes and good bacteria growth, nourishing your body with phytochemicals for cell maintenance and hormonal balance and providing antioxidants to combat free radicals. The practical way to do this is to concentrate on cleansing and rebuilding one day each week, using seeds, herbs, fruits, spices, sprouts, yogurt, and greens and other vegetables. ❧

spring for your body & mind

A day of cleansing for your body renews it like spring refreshes the natural growth of the earth. Just as a period of shedding last year's leaves makes way for fresh growth, cleansing day allows your body to remove bacteria residues and food wastes.

Most cultures recognize the need for cleansing before new growth can begin. Eastern medicine describes this process as unblocking and releasing the vital flow of energy. For overall health and high energy, all the systems of your body must work in harmony, respond to the environment, and be nourished.

Most of the cultures I have studied include cleansing as part of their health or religious practices. As a method of cleansing, some people take spring tonics and others fast. Around the world, the practice of fasting is viewed as a physical, emotional, and mental cleansing. Taking the mind off of food and allowing your body to rest from its work of digestion brings new focus to the spiritual part of life. The cleansing way is not fasting in the strictest sense, but it does allow your body a day of rest from high glycemic and stressor foods, including sugar, some animal foods, and diet foods. ❧

the cleansing way

I have created two cleansing plans to boost your immune system, to increase your energy, and to focus on harmonizing hormones, such as insulin and estrogen, through balancing the alkalinity and acidity of the foods you eat. Plan A is a program you can use once or twice a week to cleanse your body of accumulated chemicals and toxins. You can also adopt this cleansing plan as your general eating style. Plan B is a more intensive program designed to help you discover food sensitives and allergies that may be contributing to health problems.

I'll give you the plan outlines later in this chapter. First I want you to get to know the importance of the plant foods basic to cleansing your system.

ENZYMES HELP WITH DIGESTION & CLEANSING

Digestion begins in the mouth with enzymes released in saliva by the action of chewing. It continues as food travels through the gut and is broken down. Enzymes continue to work to stimulate cells to perform the chemical reactions necessary for energy, healing, digestion, and other bodily functions. The enzymes themselves do not participate in these reactions, they simply force other cells to interact with chemicals present in the bloodstream, digestive tract, and tissues. Digestive bacteria and pancreatic enzymes separate the chemical components of food and help disperse nutrients to the proper places in the body, while filtering out wastes. Enzymes are powerful, incredibly specific agents perfectly suited to the tasks they perform. Foods such as fruits, nuts, vegetables, greens, and seaweed that require chewing help stimulate enzyme production.

I often ask my patients to add extra enzyme supplements to their diets when they come to me with nutritional, environmental, psychological, hormonal, or immune system imbalance. ❧

plant foods for cleansing

Blends of leafy greens (for their chlorophyll), spiced with fresh ginger or a pinch of dried ginseng or turmeric, help to cleanse and support the liver and stimulate the gallbladder to secrete bile. Use all greens, especially cilantro, dandelion, spinach, arugula, mint, seaweed, beet leaves, and kale.

Sprouts from red clover, buckwheat, alfalfa, and beans such as garbanzos, lentils, and soybeans can be added to the leafy greens in salad, or sautéed or blended into a smoothie. Also, use root vegetables that you've steamed, sautéed, in olive oil, or roasted. There are many to choose from, such as beets, turnips, carrots, yams, sweet potatoes, and squash. To all of these, add pinches of spices, such as cumin, fennel seeds, licorice, or turmeric, and culinary herbs to balance your body's yin and yang. Fruits, especially watermelon, berries, and papaya, are highly recommended as appetizers, snacks, or desserts.

BEANS: A FOOD FOR ALL REASONS

Cooked legumes have as much calcium as milk and are also high in iron. The fiber content of legumes means they are digested more slowly and have a low glycemic index. This gives you sustained, lasting energy because eating beans doesn't result in a sudden surge of insulin. The phytochemical *saponin*, which helps to regulate insulin, is found in high amounts in legumes such as garbanzos. Legumes also can help to regulate your bowels; there are nine grams of soluble and insoluble fiber in a cup of cooked legumes. You would need to eat three to four apples to get that much fiber.

Garbanzos, delicious, heart healthy, and perhaps anticarcinogenic, are also high in isoflavones, which may lower cholesterol by as much as 35 percent (Siddiqui 1976). You can snack on celery, carrots, and cucumber sticks dipped into hummus, the popular Middle Eastern dip made from mashed garbanzo beans; baked falafel, also made from garbanzo beans, is another international favorite.

Lentils are very popular in Europe and the Middle East. They cook quickly, do not require presoaking, and have a distinctive peppery flavor. Garbanzos and lentils are both high in folic acid, an important nutrient for your heart. After flaxseeds, lentils are highest in lignan, a hormonelike substance. I recommend that you eat a cup of lentils or other beans on your cleansing day. Usually lentils do not cause you to have gas.

BERRIES: EATING COLORFULLY
FOR OUR HORMONES

I first learned about the value of berries as a small girl drinking summer tea in the Middle East, but my personal experience was confirmed on a trip I took through Russia years later. I asked a number of women from various parts of Russia to name ten foods or practices that had helped them cope with the symptoms of PMS or menopause. Every single woman I interviewed named eating different-colored berries and drinking teas made with buckwheat and berries! These results seemed especially significant, given that many Russian women live healthily into their eighties. Later, in Asia, Africa, and the Middle East, I spoke with women in their nineties and even older who also told me about brewing teas with berries of different types.

We now understand that the brightly pigmented phytohormones in brilliant red, blue, and purple berries have estrogen-like effects on the body, while their antioxidants fight infection. Berries are rich in vitamins C and E, and they help lower cholesterol levels, too. If you're looking for a quick, luxurious lift as you balance your hormones and support your endocrine system, find a way to boost your intake of fresh blueberries, blackberries, and raspberries. Both your taste buds and your hormones will thank you a hundred times over!

HEALING SEEDS FROM ALL
OVER THE WORLD

Because they absorb water, always drink whole seeds with lots of water. Some seeds absorb water from your system, and the water within the seeds also acts like a sponge, attracting and expelling substances that would normally clog your system. When swallowed whole, seeds pass through your system without leaving anything behind, like a wind blowing the leaves from a street.

Flax, psyllium, khak shir, and basil seeds are the crux of the cleansing and energy way. The fiber of these whole seeds in your system binds with cholesterol, environmental toxins, and other potentially harmful substances, and helps your body excrete them normally. These whole seeds encourage the cycle of new and healthful cell growth. They go through the entire intestinal tract, cleansing it without adding calories.

Seed Formulas

Use these seed formulas as basic drinks for cleansing and purifying your system on both plan A and plan B. ❧

shopping & preparing for cleansing

Make sure you gather the foods you need for cleansing day ahead of time. Review your health concerns in your food diary, and think about how cleansing day can help. Choose one of my two plans, or devise your own plan based on your needs. If you think you need to eliminate certain foods because of allergies or sensitivities, create a plan for the next several weeks to test for these (see cleansing plan B later in this chapter). Write down your new plan in your food wisdom diary, and then at the end of one month record the results. ❧

consider a blender

Although I don't recommend too many appliances to clutter your kitchen and believe the best way to enjoy fruits and vegetables is to chew them, many women find it convenient to use a blender. With blenders, smoothies can include nuts and seeds for essential fatty acids, vegetables, and whole fruit (pulp as well as juice).

Blending is a great way to experiment with colors and to create new combinations of flavors and textures. If you are using vegetables such as turnips, yams, pumpkins, banana squash, or sweet potatoes, steam them lightly first before blending. ❧

Sophia's Seeds Formula

Makes 3½ cups of whole seed mix, enough for 10 to 12 servings or 10 days (¼ cup or 6 tablespoons per day). You can either use all the seeds listed, or choose two or three types of seeds to get started.

1¼ cups khak shir seeds
¼ cup basil seeds
¼ cup psyllium seeds
¼ cup flaxseeds
¼ cup black sesame seeds

Mix the seeds and store them in a dry area. Organic seeds are recommended. Flax, basil, and psyllium seeds are probably the easiest to find, and the others are readily available in Middle Eastern, Chinese, and Indian food stores.

For individual servings:
¼ cup (or 4 to 6 tablespoons) Sophia's Seeds Formula
2 cups water (may use distilled water or unsweetened cranberry or other berry juices, no artificial sweetener)

Mix water and seeds together in a water bottle or other container (plastic is okay). Drink half of the mixture, including the seeds, in the morning before eating. Keep adding water to the bottle, sipping all day. (In hot climates, keep this formula refrigerated.)

Optional method I: If you do not like the gelatinous texture that forms when the seeds soak, use half of the amount of seeds, drink it down all at once, and follow with at least two glasses of plain water or sugar-free beverages. Some women prefer to just put 1 tablespoon of seeds on their tongue and swallow them whole, following this with two glasses of water. Seeds in your system without water can cause constipation, and whole seeds are not recommended if you have diverticulitis.

Optional method II: Have 2 tablespoons of seed mixture with every meal (preferably before meals). Be sure to follow this with two glasses of water. Another option is to add seeds to yogurt or pureed fruits and follow with two glasses of water. My daughter's morning joy is to mix khak shir seeds with unsweetened pomegranate juice and water.

Sophia's Seed Cooler

Add 2 tablespoons of rosewater or orange blossom water for extra phytoestrogens, and a pinch of sugar, honey, or licorice powder to seed water (you may choose only khak shir seeds). Shake it well and then drink from the bottle, including the seeds, all day. Khak shir seeds alone give excellent results.

the cleansing plans

Think of plan A as a tune-up for your body. Plan A focuses on minimizing animal foods and is more liberal than plan B, which targets specific food sensitivities and intolerances. Both plans promote lifetime wellness and longevity, boost your energy, and may help alleviate specific health symptoms.

Remember that it took you time to form the eating habits that give you the results you are experiencing now with your current diet, and it will take time to change those habits for the better.

CLEANSING PLAN A

Plan A is simply a basic model of food wisdom pyramid eating that minimizes animal food and maintains fiber and antioxidants. Plan A helps eliminate high glycemic index foods and stressor foods and emphasizes foods that help the body cleanse toxins and wastes. Concentrate on the following foods (see menus later in this chapter), eliminate any that you may be allergic to.

Foods to Eat

- Sophia's Seeds Formula

- fruits (especially assorted berries, citrus, grapes, melons, apples, pears, and pomegranates)

- greens (leafy greens and culinary herbs), sprouts (beans, seeds, and grain berries) with added spices

- vegetables, especially cruciferous vegetables, yams, seaweed, and shitake mushrooms

- Healthy and Wise Tea, Wise Flower Tea (see chapter 5 for tea recipes), Denna's Healthy Chai

- almond or sunflower seed milk, yogurt, tofu, soy milk, feta cheese, hummus, buttermilk, Sonia's Antioxidant Smoothie (see chapter 10)

- legumes, beans, seeds (especially fennel and flaxseeds), nut butters

- whole grains, brown rice, wheat germ (optional: cut out bread on your cleansing day)

- foods with omega-3 fatty acids, such as flaxseeds, walnuts, fish, and eggs

- one to two tablespoons oil per day: flaxseed oil, olive oil, sesame oil, canola oil, nut oils

- herbs and spices: tumeric, fenugreek, peppermint, red dates, licorice root, rosemary

Make Your Cleansing Day Fun

Make your day of cleansing a time to create new gastronomical delights with color and with culinary herbs and green leafy vegetables and spices. Choose recipes from this book or create your own. One young vegetarian client, Terry, chooses specific colors of plant foods to eat all day while cleansing with plan A. Some weeks, she'll eat mostly red and purple fruits and vegetables and other weeks yellow and orange. Terry tells me she has discovered a special fondness for white foods, such as cauliflower, turnips, daikon, celery, ginger, and almonds. She challenges herself to find interesting snacks in all colors and has explored how her physical feelings relate to the harmony of the foods she eats.

With each plan, I encourage conscious breathing. Oxygen is basic to the food wisdom pyramid and to the success of the healing ways and eating plans.

Schedule for One-Day-a-Week Cleansing

Choose the same day each week, if possible, so that your cleansing schedule becomes routine. Paula, an intern who claims cleansing rid her of PMS and fatigue, likes to take two days each week for cleansing and invites a friend or her sister over one weekend a month to try out new foods and recipes together. One of my students, Laura, starts each week by cleansing her body of the excess stressor foods she enjoys while socializing and traveling on weekends with friends. Mondays have become her fresh start to revive and rest her body and cleanse her liver and kidneys. Cleansing day can be whatever day best fits your lifestyle.

The following basic schedule gives you an idea of what types and combinations of food to eat during the day:

- **Mornings:** seeds (either Sophia's Seeds Formula or two to four tablespoons of mixed psyllium and flaxseeds followed by two glasses of water), smoothies, berries in different colors, grapes, pears, watermelon, culinary herbs, sprouts, leafy greens, fruit, steamed root or cruciferous vegetables with two tablespoons of vinegar.

- **Midday:** protein and vegetables (assorted greens with beans, egg, tofu, hummus, avocado, and seeds or nuts), brown rice pilaf, vegetable soup and stew, or fish.

- **Dinner:** complex carbohydrates (such as vegetables with grains), culinary herbs, sprouts, leafy greens, pilaf, vegetable stew, plain or organic yogurt with fruit.

- **All day,** drink herbal tea and water, drink some Sophia's Seeds Formula, and chew other seeds such as flaxseeds or black sesame seeds; eat fruit and vegetables for snacks.

- **Eat mindfully:** use all your senses, chew slowly, enjoy the color, taste, and fragrance of foods. Appreciate the moment and share your food with friends and colleagues.

- Take several deep breaths from the stomach before each meal.

Cleansing Day Menu Plan

This sample cleansing day menu plan gives you an idea of what and how much you will be eating.

Breakfast: seeds (one-quarter cup Sophia's Seeds Formula or flaxseeds and psyllium mixed in water or cranberry juice; or mixed leafy greens with sprouts, fresh dill and two tablespoons of flaxseeds, pears; steamed beets and yams; chai tea with soy or almond milk

Snack and tea: Healthy and Wise Tea (see chapter 5), yogurt (preferably plain and organic) topped with cantaloupe or grapes; almonds; fennel seed candies

Lunch: at a Chinese restaurant, tofu and mushroom soup; mixed vegetables (chives, ginger, eggplant, baby corn, bok choy, cabbage, broccoli, carrots) with brown rice; Sophia's Seed Formula (brought from home)

Snack and tea: carrot juice with ginger; Sonia's energizing lentil cereal; flaxseeds and sesame seeds to chew; nori seaweed sheet; soy chai latte

Dinner: Sophia's Seed Formula with two cups of distilled water; big bunch of mixed greens, tomatoes, canned garbanzo beans, radishes, and onions, with avocado, sesame seeds, with two tablespoons of balsamic vinegar, and a dash of olive oil

Before bed and tea: tea with dried figs, half a warmed yam wrapped in seaweed with yogurt

You can see that cleansing day is not about fasting but about eating as much food as you want that is colorful and balancing, packed with complex carbohydrates, antioxidants, protein, and fiber. Although you won't need to count calories, this menu plan will give you only about 1,500 to 1,900 calories a day and you can eat whenever you feel hungry. My client is also taking an organic daily supplement of multivitamins, vitamin E, calcium, vitamin D, enzymes, and vitamin C.

On this plan, start with deep breathing or meditation, then eat all the vegetables, greens, and culinary herbs you desire for any meal or snack, at any time of the day. By concentrating on legumes and fruits at meals and for snacks, you will satisfy your hunger and your body's need for nutrients. Try a Mexican-style plate of sliced tomato, onion, beans, and avocado seasoned with vinegar and salsa, or a vegetarian burrito. Your choices may be quite different from the foods listed here, but if you choose from the pyramid, they will offer you the same benefits.

Restaurant Eating on Cleansing Day

Eating in restaurants on cleansing day can be an adventure. Preparing foods at home gives you more control, but schedules don't always allow for this. If you drink your seeds formula in the morning and snack on fresh, raw vegetables, a meal in a restaurant shouldn't pose too many problems. If you go to a café, request herb tea. Perhaps the friends you're eating with will see your energy and good health and join you the next week in cleansing day, and you will all go to a juice bar instead.

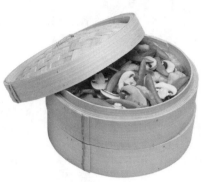

My client Gayle prefers eating in restaurants. She likes to sample food from different cultures, such as spicy bean soup in a Mexican restaurant, Chinese or Thai vegetable combinations, or Indian curries. A favorite is vegetarian burritos with beans, steamed vegetables, tomato salsa, and lettuce. If she is avoiding wheat, Gayle requests a corn tortilla and enjoys the thick, mealy texture. The jalapeño peppers, she jokes, clear her sinuses and make her eyes water, which is another form of cleansing.

Most restaurants offer vegetarian options, and you can always indulge in soups or salads. Clear soups and salads with a squeeze of lemon, your favorite vinegar, or dressing served on the side are good choices. Avoid cheese, meat, or heavy creamy sauces.

Tips for Cleansing

Remember, cleansing Plan A is only one day at a time, and only once a week unless you decide to do it more often. Nutritionally it is a balanced semivegetarian eating plan. Here are a few more tips:

- Start the day with a deep breath and an energy warmup (stretches, yoga, or qigong), and then hydrate with your seeds formula followed by two glasses of water.

- During breaks or at lunchtime, stretch, take a walk, or use some movements that incorporate conscious breathing. Gentle exercise will help your body eliminate wastes. To boost your metabolism, as well as your immune system, do not eat food for one hour after any exercise.

- Visit a juice bar for delicious blended fruits, greens, ginger, seeds, a pinch of tumeric, and vegetables.

- Create smoothies and use them on cleansing day, using color as your guide. Mix unsweetened yogurt with fresh or frozen berries, papaya, and cinnamon or ginger. Add seeds, such as flax, pumpkin, or sesame seeds, for essential fatty acids.

- Surround yourself with plants for fresh air and be thankful for their gift of beauty and oxygen.

- If you take multivitamin supplements or medications, continue taking them on cleansing day. Organic supplements, enzymes, and multivitamins are recommended.

- Let the artist within experiment with fruits and vegetables you don't eat often, such as pomegranates, papaya, kiwi, persimmon, borage, fennel, jicama, and dandelion greens.

- Add one to three tablespoons of almonds, walnuts, flaxseeds, sunflower seeds, or pumpkin seeds to salads.

- Check your color palette by checking your daily food diary for missing colors. Use cleansing day to explore foods in that color, and cover the spectrum each week. Write in your food diary.

- Eat mindfully with all your senses and take a minute to appreciate your flavorful foods and the fact you can eat in abundance from the plant world.

FOOD SENSITIVITIES

Whole foods usually are safest to eat because enzymes and nutrients are balanced in each food. In general, the body is more likely to be adapted to foods that are the simplest and most natural. There is evidence that sweets may harm insulin production and the thyroid and adrenal glands. Many food sensitivities may also be caused by digestive problems, stress, or environmental substances.

Common foods causing sensitivities or reactions include wheat, gluten products, corn, soy, citrus, yeast, eggs, refined sugar, chocolate, fish and shellfish, milk, cheese, eggplant, aspartame, saccharin, cola drinks, MSG, beef, peanuts, strawberries, onions, garlic, walnuts, chamomile, valerian, and wheatgrass. However, you can be sensitive or have a reaction to any food. Listen to your body to discover your food allergies or reactions.

Certain methods of processing, such as adding artificial color, preservatives, or fortification, may affect some people's system. If a chemical upsets the immune or digestive system, it may upset the whole body or any part of it, such as the skin, the brain (with headaches), or the lungs.

CLEANSING PLAN B

If you have food sensitivities or reactions, extreme cravings, weight gain, candida infections, or are using excess supplements, are suffering from asthma, chronic disease, or allergic reactions to environmental stress such as pollens, or are recovering from medication, illness, or infection, use plan B. It can energize you, clear your mind and respiratory passages, and may help protect your system.

Cleansing plan B allows you to experiment with your diet by introducing foods one at a time. For several days you will first eliminate foods and then reintroduce them, one by one, from least likely to cause allergies or digestive problems to those more likely to cause problems. Plan B includes all of the foods from plan A, except for wheat and any foods to which you believe you may be sensitive.

How It Works

Eliminate gluten-forming grains for three weeks. These include wheat or any flour, oats, and barley. You will reintroduce them gradually to discover your food sensitivities. If you are sensitive to wheat, you may prove sensitive to the other gluten-forming grains. While you are eliminating the gluten-forming grains, include the following gluten-free grains in your diet: brown rice, amaranth, buckwheat, quinoa, and millet. Make sure to increase other fibers such as fruits, vegetables, brown rice, and ground flaxseeds.

Step 1: Decide which other foods you would like to eliminate. Begin with

- Foods you crave; you may find these are the foods that are creating your problems.

- Foods that change your moods, making you feel euphoric, elated, or exhausted.

- Processed food, diet foods, and supplements.

- Coffee, alcohol, and tobacco.

Step 2: Pay attention to how you feel for the next three weeks. List symptoms, moods, level of energy, and other pertinent information in your food diary.

Step 3: If your major symptoms lessen or disappear, maintain step 1 for two to three months.

Step 4: Reintroduce foods you've eliminated to your diet, one by one, in small portions. Do not combine them with other foods you are limiting. If you remain symptom free, eat only that food again the next day. This gives your body time to test it. Watch for delayed responses, such as cravings, depression, mucus, bloating, or other symptoms. Then check other foods in the same way, allowing three to four days between testing each added food. Keep a record of your body's responses in your food diary.

If symptoms return with the reintroduction of any food, eliminate that food from your diet. You will know that the food that was just reintroduced should be avoided.

Raw Vegetables and Fruits

Eating many raw vegetables with cleansing plan B works well for many women who visit my clinic with chronic illnesses due to hormonal imbalance, such as heart disease and allergies, or those undergoing cancer therapy.

Biologists suggest that raw vegetables have more health benefits than cooked vegetables, in part because they contain living enzymes. You can also take organic enzyme supplements to boost the useful enzymes in your system. Cooking and heat lower or destroy some vitamins and colors of foods (freezing may also have this effect). Chinese traditional medicine believes that raw foods may deliver the electromagnetic energy that moves qi through your body and nourishes your cells.

One way to get the benefits of raw fruits and vegetables is to blend drinks to create antioxidant-rich smoothies, adding yang spices such as garlic, ginger, and pepper to balance acidity and alkalinity, but do not miss the eating fun and important digestive benefits of eating raw whole vegetables and fruits—keep cucumbers, celery, apples, jicama, and other "chewables" on hand. ❧

a few favorites

Here are a few favorites you can use on either plan:

Pomegranate is an excellent source of antioxidants. The red color feeds the heart. The combination of pomegranate and angelica (culinary spices in Middle Eastern stores) is a wonderful tonic for your blood and digestion on cleansing day. Combine one teaspoon of angelica with one tablespoon of pomegranate seeds and use as a snack or add to your tea. In some cultures, this combination is eaten to treat parasites.

Puffed amaranth makes a great snack on cleansing day, especially if you need to avoid wheat. Use a heavy pan or skillet. Cover the bottom with a layer of amaranth, and heat over medium-high heat, shaking the pan as the amaranth begins to pop. You must watch the amaranth carefully. Continue shaking and popping until all the amaranth is popped. Enjoy!

Peppermint has been a popular flavor and aroma for thousands of years. It was cultivated in monastery gardens throughout the Middle Ages in Europe and is still a favorite for kitchen gardens all over the world. The menthol from the essential oil found in peppermint leaves flavors everything from tobacco to toothpaste to mint juleps. Mint has a calming effect on the stomach and may stimulate the appetite. Use the fresh, washed leaves in salads and for cooking, as well as for tea or chewing to refresh your breath.

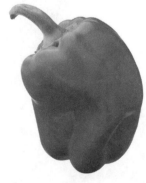

Lemon in mineral water with cucumber makes a refreshing snack on cleansing day, especially after a workout or sauna.

Sun drying eggplant is a common way to prepare this late-summer vegetable. In the Middle East, eggplants are peeled and sliced, sprinkled with salt, and spread outside under the hot sun to dry. Steam rises from the egg-plant as the liquid evaporates. Once it is dry, you can sauté onion, chopped fresh tomatoes, and eggplant in olive oil over medium heat until tender. Add a pinch of cumin seeds, turmeric, and garlic, and cook. Eggplant may have an elevating effect on moods and balance brain chemistry.

Cayenne pepper has been used for centuries to preserve and spice foods, and *capsaicin*, the active chemical, relieves pain. It benefits circulation, and the spicy qualities of cayenne may fight candida and other fungal or bacterial infections and help temporarily clear respiratory passages. Capsules are available, but why not do what Latin American and Caribbean cooks do? Use cayenne to add zing to recipes!

Ginger's properties have been much underrated in this country until recently. Because dampness was a major concern in ancient China, people depended on ginger as a major preventative and cure for illness caused by dampness and wind, its metaphoric partner. It has been considered to have anti-inflammatory and antiulcer qualities. In modern times, it is a proven preventative of motion sickness and ranks very high as a potential cancer preventative.

Fenugreek seeds are a spice that can be used fresh, powdered, or in pickling. It is an Indian and Middle Eastern folk remedy food that some people believe can help control diabetes, lower cholesterol, and keep weight balanced.

Bitter melon, or *momardica*, as it is known in Asia, Africa, and South America, is an ugly, bitter cucumber. It has been used in folk medicine as a remedy for diabetes.

chapter 4

the morning way

❧

*Make me sweet again, fragrant and
fresh and wild, and thankful for any small event.*
—Rumi

breakfast is a good place to start taking charge of your eating habits to transform your health. Your first meal of the day can be a feast for your cells, your eyes, your nose, and your brain, and can keep your insulin balanced and your body functioning at top energy all day long. Soon, you will get in the habit of looking forward to a day of healthy choices. When you wake up eager to break a long night's fast, it's important to think of food that helps you become alert and gives you energy. The morning way offers just such choices from abundant, healthy whole foods.

How does whole wheat toast topped with feta cheese, cantaloupe, walnuts, and flaxseeds, accompanied by mint tea, sound for breakfast? If you were a woman living in the eastern Mediterranean, this would be a typical breakfast. Or you might opt to eat steamed beets with a sprinkling of sesame seeds, or perhaps ricotta cheese with tomatoes and fresh basil on whole grain bread, or dried figs and almonds. In China, women wake up to enjoy green tea and a bowl of warm fresh soy milk and rice, adding diced foods to the rice to vary the taste. This chapter offers food menus and recipes to help you make breakfast nutritious and flexible.

the first food of the day

Breakfast is the most important meal of the day. A breakfast of high-fiber foods balances insulin, contributes to regularity, reduces cravings, helps eliminate wastes, and makes room in your digestive tract for new foods to provide energy. In addition to physical energy, breakfast provides the nourishment your brain needs for mental activity and concentration.

Eating complex carbohydrates in the morning provides a steady release of insulin and the neurotransmitter serotonin all day, for balanced, calm moods, good mental acuity, and healthy weight. Complex carbohydrates, protein, and phytochemicals—the elements I suggest for breakfast —are the best line of defense against hormonal imbalance and disease.

ARE YOU SKIPPING BREAKFAST?

Your body needs steady energy throughout the day. If you skip breakfast, you probably feel low energy or experience fatigue in the afternoon and later in the day. If you don't eat breakfast, your metabolism may slow down to compensate for not receiving any new calories. A study by Dr. C. Wayne Callaway (1987) found that people who eat breakfast burn more calories throughout the day than people who skip it. I have seen this fact demonstrated with clients who came to me with digestive difficulties. One client told me she skipped breakfast because she usually wasn't hungry until noon and she was trying to lose weight. She wasn't losing weight, however, but was often constipated and experienced cravings for sweets in the evening. When she made a healthy breakfast part of her day, she was better able to maintain her diet.

UNDERSTANDING YOUR CURRENT HABITS

One thing I have learned from working with women over the years is that before you can make a change in your eating habits for the better, you need to know what you want to change and what you are already doing that works for you. Marion, who came to me with irritable bowel syndrome and fatigue, never ate breakfast, always rushing out the door each day. She agreed to change her pattern by having fruit and grains in the morning and taking the time for deep breathing. Her symptoms disappeared and she looks forward to her morning repast while watching the sunrise. "I feel as though I am eating the colors in the sky," she said.

Take a minute to answer the following questions in your food diary. Look over what you've eaten in the morning over the last few days, or think about your usual patterns.

- *What did you eat for breakfast today?*

- *Do you often skip breakfast? How do you feel later in the afternoon?*

- *What do you normally eat for breakfast?*

- *What are your normal activities?*

- *Do you have energy in the afternoon?*

- *Can you remember your mood after eating breakfast?*

- *What about your mood in the late morning if you skip breakfast?*

- *Are you often constipated?*

- *Do you often have diarrhea?*

- *Do you have at least one or two bowel movements a day?*

- *Do you strain to move your bowels?*

- *Have you ever had gastrointestinal problems, such as irritable bowel syndrome, diverticulitis, or gastroesophageal reflux?*

- *What would you like to change about your current breakfast eating habits, or are you happy with them?*

- *What would you like to change about your current moods in the late morning and afternoon, or are you happy with them?*

- *Do you have any specific health problems that you would like to improve?*

WHAT YOU NEED TO FUEL YOUR DAY

The way to fuel your body for the day to come is to eat a breakfast that combines essential elements from the food pyramid: fiber, protein, essential fat, antioxidants, and complex carbohydrates. Each morning, make taking a few deep breaths a part of your routine because none of the foods you eat will work as well for your body without a strong supply of oxygen. Perhaps you'll make your tea and sit with it, breathing deeply, before leaving for work or during breakfast. Sit in front of a window, watching the sky, to help feel a part of the beautiful natural world. Or, just breathe in deeply a few times before rising from bed. Hydrate yourself with water and with your tea, or with your seeds in water, if it is a cleansing day. In addition to these nutritional needs, don't neglect your spiritual and emotional needs. If you can make time to write in your journal or meditate each morning, you'll be rewarded with peace of mind and energy all day. ❧

fiber breakfast for healthy digestion & daylong energy

What you eat for breakfast can have a profound effect on your feeling of comfort, your stress level, and your bowel regularity. News reports and health organizations advise Americans to eat more fiber. The FDA recommends a fiber intake of 20 to 35 grams a day, yet many women get only half of that or less. Just knowing the importance of fiber doesn't mean you'll eat more. In this chapter, you'll learn an easy way to incorporate fiber into your lifestyle and how to create delicious hot or cold grain and lentil cereals, healthy take-along energy shakes, fruity muffins, vegetable omelets, and more.

Simple carbohydrates are starch and sugar without fiber. With fiber, they become complex carbohydrates. Complex carbohydrates are found in whole grain breads and cereals, herbs, vegetables, fruits, nuts, seeds, and legumes. These whole foods are alive with phytochemicals, vibrant colors, textures, aromas, and flavors, making them a pleasure to eat. Complex carbohydrates are rich in vitamins, minerals, and antioxidants.

Fiber is not digested but it influences the way your body uses other nutrients. Fiber aids digestion and can prevent constipation and other gastrointestinal problems, and it may lower cholesterol, prevent adverse hormonal symptoms, and prevent cancer. As it passes through the digestive tract, fiber is the bulk that keeps everything moving along with it, especially waste products.

Here's a fun recipe to help give you the fiber you need to start your day. ❧

Silky Fruity Muffins

MAKES 8–12 LARGE MUFFINS

Breakfast won't seem so dull when you have these flavor-packed morsels to bite into. Serve with tea or chai latte, or coffee spiked with cinnamon.

> 1¼ cups oat bran
> 1 cup wheat bran
> 1 teaspoon baking powder
> ¼ teaspoon salt (optional)
> ¼ cup chopped walnuts (optional)
> 4 eggs (or 8 egg whites)
> ½ cup berries, such as raspberries, currants, cherries, cranberries, blueberries (optional)
> ¼ cup orange juice
> 1 tablespoon honey or molasses
> 4 dates, chopped (optional)
> 1 medium banana, mashed
> 1 tablespoon grated orange zest
> 1 tablespoon liquid vegetable oil or light olive oil

Preheat the oven to 425°F. Combine the dry ingredients.

In another bowl, combine the wet ingredients, and add them to the dry. Stir just to mix. Pour the mixture into nonstick muffin pans and bake 14 to 17 minutes.

Variations: *Substitute 1 ounce soft tofu, pureed, for eggs. Substitute pecans, pistachios, or sesame seeds for the walnuts.*

a colorful rainbow of phytochemicals

Choosing fresh, colorful, seasonal fruit for breakfast can be a part of your food artistry. You might consider finding organic fruit, to avoid soil and pesticide contaminants, but remember to choose fresh fruit that is in season because it will contain more nutrients and no preservatives. Fruits are important for their fiber, antioxidants, and vitamins.

My personal choice for breakfast is an Asian pear, which is a low glycemic index food that contains high fiber and is low in acidity. For vegetarians, whose diets are high in alkalinity, grapefruit may aid digestion by adding acidic properties. Citrus fruits offer vitamins C and A, and beta-carotene, but may cause stomach upset in some individuals because they are high in acid. Melons offer an excellent balance of antioxidants, minerals, and vitamins, high fiber, a refreshing taste, and low 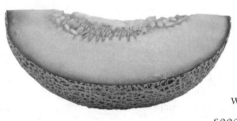 acidity; eating them with nuts and seeds will balance your acidity and alkalinity. Bananas provide potassium in addition to other nutrients. Chinese and Persian medical practitioners recommend that you balance bananas (considered a "hot" food) with "cool" foods such as cilantro, anise seeds, or melon. Apples are another great choice, and with the many varieties now available, you could eat a different type of apple each day for your apple a day, and not repeat for a couple of weeks! Cherries, strawberries, raspberries, pomegranates, and blueberries are phytoestrogenic and good antioxidant choices, and can be used throughout the year in frozen or dried forms or in juices. Dried fruits, such as figs, raisins, dates, and apricots, can add variety during the winter months.

As a food artist, combine and contrast: choose different fruits in different colors throughout the week and the seasons to go with what appeals to you and to provide a variety of phytonutrients and other nutrients. Follow your nose and eyes as you pick different varieties throughout the week, engaging your senses to feed your body different nutrients. Choose orange fruits one day and red or green the next. Balance dark red beets with creamy yogurt. Add crunchy nuts to your chewy oatmeal as a treat for your mouth. Shakes combining yogurt and fruit make a quick convenient breakfast. You can try them in a variety of color combinations, adding fruit as you choose. ❧

MAKES 2 SHAKES

2 eggs or 3 egg whites, or ½ cup egg substitute, or 2 teaspoons dried egg powder, and/or 2 tablespoons soy protein or garbanzo flour

¼ cup soft tofu or ½ cup plain yogurt, or a combination

2 tablespoons grains, such as oat, rice bran, or cereal (optional)

I tablespoon flaxseeds or almonds, or any nuts, seeds, or oil, such as walnut, you feel you need therapeutically (ground, paste, or whole)

I teaspoon honey (optional) or ¼ cup frozen orange juice concentrate

I cup fresh raspberries or other berries of your choice

Sprig of fresh mint, a cinnamon stick, or nutmeg for garnish

Coddle whole eggs in their shells by placing them in boiling water for 2 minutes. If you prefer, you can cook the eggs for 3 minutes and use the white only. (You can do several eggs at once to this stage and store in the refrigerator for up to one week for later use.)

Peel or crack the eggs. If not using the yolks, separate and save the yolks for another use.

Combine all the ingredients except garnish and blend for 3 minutes in a blender.

Garnish with a sprig of mint, a cinnamon stick, or a dusting of freshly grated nutmeg.

Variations: *Add one or more of these fruits to the basic shake and blend for an additional 10 to 15 seconds: ¼ cup fresh or frozen berries (without added sugar, if possible); ¼ cup diced fresh or canned pear; quarter banana with 2 drops of vanilla and a dash of cardamom; ¼ cup diced papaya; 1 small orange, diced and with seeds removed; ¼ cup fresh or canned chopped peaches; half a medium apple (diced) and 2 drops rosewater (optional); 1 large kiwi, peeled.*

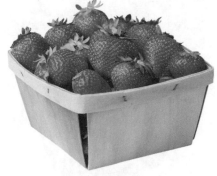

If you also are using juice, add a juice that matches the fruit you chose, such as apple juice with apple or pineapple juice with pineapple.

plant protein for bright mornings & alert days

Proteins are called the building blocks of our bodies and we need protein to start our day with power and energy. Protein is of primary importance to the body and you should eat it first thing in the morning.

Protein provides the essential amino acids for the body to perform its work each day. My morning way menus, based on the multicultural food wisdom pyramid, emphasize a variety of plant foods that provides complete plant protein.

Adding whole grains and nuts to yogurt, cereal, smoothies, or snacks will provide complete protein, as will adding garbanzo flour, amaranth, soy, or tofu. Again, variety is the key. As you learn to plan ahead for easy, healthy eating, you'll discover new combinations to feed your needs and your appetite. As you slowly incorporate some of these breakfast

Egg Foo Yong (Chinese Omelet)

MAKES 4–6 SERVINGS

Morning protein will keep you alert with the help of antioxidants. This omelet is packed with flavor and the tofu and mushrooms give it a meaty texture. Leftovers of this Asian frittata make great brown-bag lunches.

> **2 cups firmed tofu, drained and diced**
> **6 eggs, lightly beaten**
> **1 cup each: sliced mushrooms; seeded and chopped red pepper; chopped green onions; and bean sprouts**
> **1 teaspoon soy sauce**
> **Black pepper to taste**
> **Assorted greens, for garnish**

Preheat the oven to 350°F.

Combine the tofu and eggs, stir in the remaining ingredients except greens, and pour into a greased baking dish.

Bake for 20 minutes or until lightly browned. Allow to cool before cutting.

Divide the greens between serving plates or place on a large serving platter. Place the frittata on the greens and serve at room temperature.

Variations: *Egg Foo Yong Patties: Heat 2 tablespoons oil in a pan on the stovetop and spoon the frittata mixture into the hot oil. Sauté until golden brown on both sides. Serve on bed of greens or on whole grain hamburger buns or in pita pockets. Substitute chopped cooked chicken, beef, pork, or ham for the tofu, or add with the tofu. Seafood Foo Yong: Substitute 6 ounces of cooked, peeled shrimp for the tofu.*

choices into your life, you'll notice changes in the way you feel and higher levels of energy. Keep track of which proteins worked best for you prior to a day of physical activity or an important meeting. If you have particular health concerns, adjust your protein, fiber, and phytochemicals accordingly. (See chapter 8.)

You don't need to use formulas to determine which proteins are complete. Eating a variety of colors, textures, and aromas throughout the week will balance your protein intake. If you prefer something crunchy some mornings, opt for chewy nuts with bread. With all these flavorful—and healthful—options, you can say good-bye to boring breakfasts. 🎍

Pistachio Tofu Pudding

MAKES I SERVING

This festive, beautiful pudding is a perfect brunch choice, especially served in crystal glasses and garnished with fresh blackberries. Just increase the recipe to serve a number of guests.

3 to 5 ounces tofu (silken or soft works best)
½ cup berries, fresh or frozen
¼ cup shelled pistachios
I cup almond, rice, or soy milk
Powdered pistachio, for garnish
Sprig of fresh mint, for garnish

Blend the tofu, berries, pistachios, and milk and serve in a crystal glass or pottery bowl, depending on your mood. Garnish with powdered pistachio and fresh mint.

variety through grains

Besides being delicious, inexpensive, abundant, and versatile, grains are a great source of complex carbohydrates, fiber, phytochemicals, and protein. Whole grains are the dietary foundation of some of the healthiest cultures in the world. The easiest way to eat grains is in cereal, and many Americans already eat cereal for breakfast. Foods rich in fiber, phytoestrogen, chromium, niacin, magnesium, and essential fatty acids keep your blood sugar balanced and steady. You can achieve this balance by cooking whole grains such as brown rice or bulgur with greens, by using Sonia's Phytoestrogenic Cereal Formula, or by adapting some of the following ideas.

Sonia's Energizing Lentil Cereal

MAKES 6–8 SERVINGS

The angelica in this recipe is great for digestion and may help prevent the gas some people experience when they aren't used to eating legumes. Anise and fenugreek (a favorite for digestion in Afghan cuisine) or cardamom can be substituted with the same result. This is an excellent recipe for cleansing day or for those with a sensitivity to grains.

I cook this excellent source of complete protein on Sunday and keep it all week. My children heat it each morning for about 1 minute. My athletic son always eats this, his favorite dish, before competitions, claiming it helps his endurance and keeps his energy up.

You won't go away hungry after indulging in this hot and savory cereal. If you don't soak the lentils ahead of time, add about 20 minutes to the cooking time. Soaked lentils will create a thicker base.

1 pound French lentils or any lentil you prefer

2 medium red onions, chopped

3 to 5 cloves garlic, minced (optional)

1 teaspoon fresh ginger, minced (optional)

1 teaspoon each turmeric, ground cumin seed, and curry powder

3 tablespoons olive oil

1 tablespoon oatmeal or barley (optional)

salt and pepper to taste

2 to 3 lemons, halved, for garnish

1 tablespoon angelica, for garnish

Soak the lentils overnight in 2 quarts water

Bring the lentils and soaking water to boil. Reduce the heat and cook for 40 to 45 minutes, or until tender.

Sauté the onions, garlic, ginger, and spices in the oil for 10 minutes. Add to the cooked lentils and mix well.

Mix the oatmeal and a little warm water to make a smooth paste. Add to the lentil mixture, mix well, and cook over medium heat, stirring, until it looks like hot cereal. This should be about 5 minutes.

Serve with a half lemon (for squeezing in the juice) and a sprinkle of angelica.

Menu suggestion: *Accompany with crisp bread, herbed yogurt, nuts, or flaxseeds. Serving with cantaloupe and grapes will provide a great breakfast and balance the body.*

In Russia, your breakfast bowl might contain buckwheat, almonds, berries, and raisins. In Asia, rice noodles and tofu would be central ingredients. Africans and Middle Easterners eat breakfasts of hot lentils or black beans with cumin, angelica, feta cheese, and grapes. In the Middle East, a typical steaming bowl of cereal would include a variety of grains, legumes, and spices. In Turkey, sprouted wheat and beans are popular and satisfying choices.

BOXED CEREAL CAN BE A HEALTHY BEGINNING

The fiber content of most boxed cereal ranges from half a gram to fourteen grams, so read the labels carefully, and choose cereal with high fiber content. Boxed whole grain and corn cereals can be useful nutritionally, especially when you add a variety of fruits, nuts and seeds. Try these new approaches to adding variety, balance, and nutrition to eating cereal:

- Skip sugar and add fresh and dried fruit to sweeten cereal naturally.

- Add seeds and nuts, especially almonds, sesame seeds, walnuts, flaxseeds, and spices, for extra fiber, texture, and taste.

- Try almond milk or soy milk fortified with calcium, instead of cow's milk. Soy, rice, and nut milks don't contain saturated fat or the hormones and antibiotics given to animals, and they are high in complex carbohydrates, fiber, vitamins, and minerals.

- Look for amarath, psyllium, flaxseed, or rice bran cereals. They are an excellent source of soluble

Homemade Granola

MAKES 5 CUPS

This recipe provides plenty of nutrition and good flavor with less fat and sugar than traditional versions. It makes a good and fast cereal, meal, or snack any time of day.

> **I cup raw wheat germ**
> **I cup rolled oats or flaxseeds**
> **I tablespoon cashews, chopped**
> **¼ cup almonds, chopped or slivered**
> **¼ cup sunflower seeds**
> **¼ cup raisins**
> **I tablespoon sesame oil**
> **I tablespoon brown sugar**
> **I tablespoon honey**
> **I tablespoon orange zest**

Preheat the oven to 375°F

Mix all the ingredients together well and bake for 15 to 20 minutes, or until desired doneness. Serve at once, with low-fat milk and fresh fruit, or store in a tightly sealed jar in the refrigerator for up to 2 months.

Variations*: Top with plain yogurt and garnish with berries or mint. Fill half a cantaloupe with granola and cottage cheese. For barley granola, substitute barley bran for the rolled oats.*

Sonia's Phytoestrogenic Cereal Formula

MAKES 5 CUPS

This phytoestrogenic cereal formula includes high protein, calcium, boron, isoflavones, and fiber and phytoestrogenic properties. This recipe makes about enough for a week or two, but it can be made in larger batches and frozen. Using this entire list of ingredients is the ideal goal, but even if you choose only four of the ingredients and add them to your favorite packaged cereal, you've made a promising nutritional start. Make shopping for grains a monthly task, and freeze cereal for convenience.

Ingredients: ¼ cup of each of the following:

- **Amaranth**
- **Chopped dried apricots**
- **Ground buckwheat**
- **Flaxseeds**
- **Quinoa, triticale, berries (such as cranberries, cherries or currants)**
- **Wheat flakes, sunflower seeds, and rye flakes**
- **Chopped almonds or barley flakes**
- **Rice bran, rolled oats, raisins, or chopped dates**
- **Orange zest**
- **Pinch of cinnamon or cardamom**
- **Dash of honey or maple syrup (optional)**

Mix together, keep in a glass jar or bottle, and refrigerate.

Microwave: *You may also cook a ½ cup portion of mixed cereal with liquid in the microwave on medium power for 2 to 4 minutes. Try adding a sliced apple with 1 cup of almond milk or berry juice and cook.*

Stovetop: *In a saucepan, combine 1 cup of cereal with 2 cups of liquid. Try milk, soy milk, rice milk, nut milk, juice, or water. Bring to a boil and cook, stirring, for 5 to 10 minutes or until it reaches the consistency you prefer. For a softer consistency and faster cooking, soak the cereal for an hour in the liquid before cooking.*

Served cold: *Serve cooked cereal at room temperature mixed with milk, soy milk, rice milk, almond milk, or any juice (fruit or vegetable, such as apple or carrot juice). If desired, add other favorite cereals, as much as you want, to your taste.*

fiber and phytohormones, which help to lower cholesterol and keep blood sugar in balance. Foods to add to what you're already eating for breakfast that will raise fiber and phytohormone intake include psyllium seeds, prunes, figs, rice bran, oat bran, and wheat germ. ❧

root vegetables

Eating root vegetables can be a delicious and colorful way to start your day. Drawing minerals and vitamins and other nutrients from the earth is the job of root vegetables, and these healing foods are some of my favorite breakfast choices from Mother Nature's kitchen.

Turnips, celery, radishes, parsnips, and carrots are delicious raw, but you can also use them cooked. Brightly colored beets, sweet potatoes, potatoes, and yams can be baked or roasted ahead of time for quick and easy take-along breakfasts packed with fiber and nutrients. One medium sweet potato provides 520 percent of your daily requirement of vitamin A and 50 percent of vitamin C, and has only 140 calories (if you don't add fats or sweets).

In Mexico, Europe, and the Middle East, people eat turnips when they feel a cold or sore throat coming on. These cultures believe turnips may have an antibiotic effect. More scientific research is needed into some of this cultural wisdom, but I have had the experience of using turnips in this therapeutic way in my practice for several years, with excellent results. Women in many cultures also eat sweet potatoes for balance and beets for cleansing.

We've all enjoyed home-fried potatoes or hash browns with breakfast in a restaurant, but have you ever considered pan-frying slices of baked sweet potato? Simply use a little olive oil over medium heat in a heavy skillet to sauté them. Sprinkle them with herbs and spices such as cinnamon, ginger, anise, dill, and angelica to add more nutrients, flavor, and variety.

COOKING ROOT VEGETABLES

You can make several of these at one time and have a supply for the entire week. Vegetables to bake, microwave, or steam include potatoes (buy yellow, creamy potatoes, such as Yellow Finns or Yukon golds), beets, turnips, sweet potatoes, and yams.

Baking is best for root vegetables. You can bake or cook several varieties at the same time. Wash but don't peel them. Leave the vegetables whole. Bake at 375°F for 35 to 45 minutes. Large yams will take longer. If you plan to heat them in a microwave later, you may not need to cook them as long. (As an alternative, add about an inch of water to a pan and bring to boil. Add the vegetables in a steamer basket, cover, and cook until they reach the desired level of doneness; you may need to add more water during cooking.) According to Chinese medicine, eating these foods at room temperature is best for your digestive system, but if you prefer them warm, reheat before eating.

One or one and a half of these vegetables for breakfast makes a good serving size. Or, slice them and mix or match. Root vegetables have strong, delicious flavors without added seasoning, so you can try them just as they are or, for variety, eat with crushed seaweed, yogurt, vinegar, herbs, lemon, lime, or chopped green onion. Suggested seasonings are oregano, chives, basil, pepper, turmeric, cumin, crushed flaxseeds, fennel seeds, cayenne pepper, and grated ginger. ❧

putting your morning way plan into action

I hope this chapter has inspired you to begin enjoying breakfast more. You can find more recipes for the morning way in chapter 10. Now, it is time to plan how you will put together a breakfast to strengthen your own body and maintain high energy throughout the day. Set small goals first, and over time your choices will begin to include a wider variety of plant foods for your fiber- and protein-rich breakfasts.

To make it easy, you can prepare your food the night before and leave it out of the refrigerator. The food will at be room temperature, the best for eating, or ready to warm up, in the morning.

YOUR PERSONAL BREAKFAST PLAN

Now set a goal for your personal breakfast plan that you will follow over the next few weeks. Go back to the questionnaire at the beginning of this chapter. Perhaps you'll use one of my menu plans (see the next section in this chapter) two or three times a week, and the rest of the week eat your usual breakfast of cereal, adding raisins and fresh fruit, or eat a bagel with almond butter and jam, feta cheese, or hummus, sprinkled with nuts and flaxseeds. Keep track of your goals, and how you feel each day, in your food diary. As you feel better, you'll find it easier to eat a healthy breakfast.

Here are a few key points to remember about eating breakfast:

- Begin the day with oxygen by taking deep breaths and breathing in the aroma of your tea or coffee.

- Breakfast is the fuel for your day, and is the best way to keep your insulin and glucose levels and metabolism balanced for steady energy.

- Protein and fiber in the form of complex carbohydrates should be part of your breakfast.

- Balance nutrients by choosing a variety of colorful and flavorful seeds, culinary herbs, fruits, root vegetables, whole grains, and nuts for breakfast.

- Breakfast can be fast and easy, especially with planning and preparing several foods at a time for eating later in the week.

Based on these reminders, set three goals for yourself for the coming week. Here are some sample goals:

- "Once this week, I'll eat root vegetables for breakfast that I bake the night before with my dinner."

- "I'll keep flaxseeds mixed with black sesame seeds in my purse, at my desk, or in my car in case I'm running late or still feel hungry. I'll eat them with fruit or a muffin."

- "This week, I'll shop for whole grains to make a batch of cereal for freezing and eating. I'll eat the cereal three mornings this week."

- "Two days this week, I'll eat a bunch of grapes or a pear. I'll think about their different texture and taste and how I feel when I eat them."

- "This weekend, I'll make lentil cereal or a Chinese tofu omelet for breakfast."

LIFESTYLE SUGGESTIONS FOR THE MORNING

Start each day with a morning stretch. Use tai chi temple exercises, yoga sun salutation, dance warmup routines, runner's stretches, or qigong movements to start your day. All of these are simple to learn, and you can find instructions in many books or through community classes. Qigong and tai chi are now offered in many outdoor parks throughout the United States, and videotapes are availabe for practice at home.

At work, relieve stress with a five-minute break: stretch your neck and shoulder muscles by slowly making circles with your head; visualize a peaceful scene; or practice progressive muscle relaxation. You can do any of these things right at your desk, or anywhere else you find yourself in need of stress relief.

MENU SUGGESTIONS FOR THE MORNING

These suggestions will balance your weekly intake of protein, nutrients, and non-nutrients, such as fiber and phytohormones, while providing choice and variety. Drink a cup of tea along with these foods.

1. Sonia's Phytoestrogenic Cereal

two slices of watermelon

❧

2. cereal (buckwheat, amaranth, oat, or quinoa) with soy milk or yogurt, honey, grapes, and dried apricots

❧

3. Sonia's Energizing Lentil Cereal sprinkled with marjoram, angelica, or ground sesame seeds

toasted whole grain raisin bread

papaya with lemon

❧

4. vegetable-filled omelet

baked potato

pomegranate juice

❧

5. two roasted beets

whole grain seeded bagel with goat, ricotta, or cream cheese

warmed almond milk

❧

6. roasted, steamed, or microwaved yam, turnip and/or sweet potato

rye toast

chapter 5

tea, oxygen, & movement

We drank tea on the meadow of the table,
I opened the door: a piece of sky fell into my glass.
But no, I was out for the stars;
I drank the sky down with the tea.
—Sohrab Sepehri

the top of the food wisdom pyramid is sunlight, oxygen, water, and tea (with its myriad spices and diverse plant foods). These are our most essential needs. Tea combines many different types of herbs, spices, and other plants, bringing the goodness of the earth to your body. Coffee comes from only one plant, so it is less diverse and has fewer health benefits.

Oxygen is the element that powers the use of food through digestion, helps the mind function, and helps nourish every cell and muscle. When you drink water, your body is properly hydrated. Tea made in the way described in this book gives aroma, color, taste, and added nutrients, fiber, and phytohormones. It helps you regulate the water you need for your body, eliminate wastes, cleanse your systems, or retain fluids as needed, according to the ingredients you use. ❧

tea: bridging east & west

Green and black teas are one of the oldest and most valued beverages in the world. In China, green and black teas have been used for cleansing and medicinal purposes for over four thousand years. Tea is widely appreciated for its delicate flavor and fragrance and for the sense of calm and spirituality that it can provide.

In many cultures, tea is used not only to promote physical health, but as a social institution. In Russia, for example, families believe that a house without a samovar is a house without a foundation.

In America, the observance of an English or Asian teatime has become an increasingly popular trend. Oriental tea gardens, tea houses, and English-style tea shops have grown up around the idea of tea as ceremony—complete with fresh sliced cucumber on tiny triangles of bread or the good, country taste of a Scottish scone, to which you treat a grandchild, mother, or friend.

Sonia's Tea for Life

Each of the ingredients in this tea has been selected for pigment, hormonal qualities, and flavor. You can also add a tea bag of your choice, such as black currant or plum. There are numerous ingredients listed, so pick and choose what you prefer, what you can find at the store, or what you have on hand. To prepare the tea, mix all the ingredients and keep in a tightly sealed jar until ready to use.

I tablespoon of one or more of the following: cardamom seeds, crushed cinnamon, savory, sage, anise seeds, fennel seeds, sweet fennel, dill seeds, dried apricot, dried apple, hibiscus flower, rooibos or red tea, ginseng, rose hips, diced licorice, any dried berries, orange zest, roasted brown rice

½ cup of one or more of the following tea leaves: green or black tea, borage, mint, jasmine tea, sencha, bancha green tea, genmaicha, Darjeeling tea, Ceylon tea, other tea leaves available in the market

Select any combination of these ingredients or mix all of them together. Omit any ingredients you have an allergy to. Store the blend in a lidded large glass jar. Keeps indefinitely. To prepare for serving, add hot water to I tablespoon of mixed tea and let steep for 2 to 4 minutes. Then strain and enjoy sipping. Dilute with hot water as desired.

RESEARCH SUPPORTS THE USE
OF TEA FOR HEALTH

Research is now showing that many cultural habits, practices, and beliefs, after centuries of use, are rooted in actual health benefits. Tea contains some powerful phytochemicals: a group of antioxidants called *polyphenols*. Researchers suspect that one type of polyphenol found in tea, called *catechins*, is useful in removing toxins in the body to protect us from cancer. They also may reduce *hypolipidemia* (excess fat levels in the blood), and reduce the risk for hypertension by lowering fat levels in the blood. Some scientific studies credit tea, that is, the leaves of the tea plant processed as black or green tea, with a variety of possible therapeutic benefits. These studies indicate tea may

- improve functioning of the immune system

- reduce risk of heart disease and of certain cancers

- fight infections and bacterial diarrhea

- lower blood pressure

- prevent cavities, due to fluorine content

Denna's Herbal Chai

A red, sweet cupful of Herbal Chai includes the exotically refreshing taste of the South African Rooibos plant, a sweet herb overflowing with antioxidants for releasing energy, balancing the body's Yin and Yang properties, easing anxiety, and balancing blood sugar. Adored for its harmonizing qualities as preparation for Zen meditation, this delightful mixture blends the zing of pepper and allspice with the sweet surprise of nutmeg, ginger, and licorice for an amazingly balanced flavor, which encourages healthy enjoyment and aids digestion. Caffeine free, Herbal Chai is excellent as a latte, with soy or almond milk.

Combine I tablespoon of each ingredient:
- **Ginger (root or powdered)**
- **Rooibos**
- **Powdered or chopped licorice root**
- **Orange peel**

½ tablespoon of the following ingredients:
- **Cayenne pepper**
- **black pepper**
- **Fennel**
- **Coriander**
- **Nutmeg**
- **Allspice**

Mix I tablespoon of the tea in a cup of hot water or in your tea infuser.

When I placed tea in my food wisdom model, I was thinking about its main health benefit as a great comfort food and health snack.

Tea can be as simple as pouring hot water over the fresh mint leaves you just snipped from your garden. Tea bags, of course, are so easy to use, and come bearing so many different flavors of tea. Think of tea as a fun nutrition vehicle to help you add spices, culinary herbs, roasted grains, seeds, and dried fruits to your diet. You will be in good company since many of the women I have observed abroad depend on fresh teas to maintain equilibrium, soothe menstrual cramps, and keep hydrated.

CHOOSE YOUR FAVORITE COLOR: GREEN OR BLACK

People frequently wonder whether black or green tea provides the most benefits. Both are excellent sources for catechins, but green tea contains more. Green tea is steamed, then immediately rolled and dried. Black tea is crushed and left to ferment. This process of oxidation gives the tea its dark color. We're not sure what effects the oxidation process has on the benefits of tea, beyond lowering the levels of polyphenols. In the finished product, black tea has about 35 to 75 milligrams of catechins per dry gram, while green tea has 80 to 180 milligrams.

For this reason, many experts recommend green tea. Studies have shown, however, that while cancer levels are low among tea-drinking populations in Japan and China, where green tea is common, the same is true of tea drinkers in the Middle East and the Mediterranean, where black tea is preferred. You can feel good about drinking either, but make sure to include some green tea.

You can increase the natural phytoestrogenic benefits of your tea by adding spices, culinary herbs, and fruits, such as chopped apple, dill, mint, ginger, and fennel seeds. Russian women add fresh or dried berries to their tea to lessen menopausal discomforts. Women in the Middle East add cherries, borage, and lemon.

PRACTICAL TEA TIPS

- I've noted that plain, strong tea can have undesirable side effects on some people, affecting their digestion or causing them to feel edgy. Several cups of tea a day can be constipating

Wise Flower Tea

MAKES 5 – 7 CUPS.

Combine I teaspoon of each ingredient:

- **green tea leaves**
- **rooibos**
- **ginseng**
- **lavender**
- **crushed rose hips**
- **chrysanthemum petals (optional)**
- **hibiscus flower (optional)**

Mix all the ingredients together. Store in an airtight container. Use I teaspoon for each cup of tea.

or a diuretic, depending on individual digestive systems and other physiological balances.

- People of some ethnic groups have learned to avoid unpleasant side effects by adding rose leaves, cardamom, clove, ginger, mint, cinnamon, and other culinary herbs, spices, and flavorings to water along with a little tea. The tea recipes in this book are designed to minimize caffeine and tannic acid, too much of which can cause problems with digestion, jitteriness, and insomnia.

- The oxidation process used in producing black tea may reduce the body's ability to absorb iron. For menopausal women, however, this may be a positive side effect; according to a Finnish study, excess levels of iron can increase the risk of heart disease. For any young woman or perimenopausal woman who is susceptible to iron deficiencies, drinking herbal or fruit tea is the wise choice. Adding fresh lemon or lime juice, which contains the antioxidant vitamin C, to black tea may increase iron absorption and provide a delicious flavor.

- Try drinking your tea out of a clear glass, so that you can make sure it is well diluted and light in color. If you use a tea bag to make your tea, dip it in a few times and then remove it. In cultures where tea is a common beverage, people know drinking strong tea can also stain the teeth. They brush their teeth with baking soda or salt to remove these stains. You can speak to your dentist about other effective stain removal techniques if staining occurs. Green tea, especially, protects from the growth of *Streptococcus Mutans*, the bacteria causing cavities and gingivitis, because it contains the polyphenol epigallocatechin gallate (EGCG). The enzyme urokinase, which feeds tumors that grow by destroying the protein of normal cells, is also blocked by EGCG (Fujiki et al. 2003).

- Have fun shopping in ethnic markets where ingredients for tea can be bought separately. Mix and make your own teas; buy in bulk and keep them in a big jar. Remember, you pay for packaging, although you may like to collect pretty tea boxes and tins for which you can also find other uses.

- When buying bottled iced tea, choose ones without artificial sweeteners or additives, and with natural fruit flavorings. Keep in mind that sweetened iced tea can contain up to 180 calories in a bottle. If you're concerned about calories, make your own iced tea, or buy unsweetened ready-made tea. Reward yourself with a nice teapot, so that you can consider every tea encounter a treat.

- Tea is also a wonderful aid when you increase fiber in your diet. After a meal of plant foods such as beans and legumes, drink some tea with honey and cardamom. This tasty mixture will help you avoid mild indigestion and the gas problems that high fiber intake can sometimes cause.

HERBAL TEA

There is a difference between herbal medicine and herbal teas. Some people have allergic reactions to chamomile and other herbs. If you determine that you have no adverse reactions, then you may benefit from the phytoestrogenic

Healthy & Wise Tea

MAKES 15 TO 18 CUPS
This formula is hormonally harmonized to be a woman's strengthening and balancing tea.

   2 tablespoons each green tea and damiana leaves
   4 to 5 each red clover flowers and cardamom seeds
   2 tablespoons rooibos leaves
   I teaspoon each fennel seeds, crushed rose hips and petals, hibiscus petals, barberries, chrysanthemum petals, and black tea (optional)

Mix everything together. Steep in a teapot for all-day use or use I teaspoon at a time for each cup of tea.

Variation: *A pinch of black cohosh and angelica or dong quai can be substituted for hibiscus.*

properties of herb, spice, and fruit-flavored teas. These may contain a variety of hormonal plants such as chamomile, ginseng, borage, and culinary herbs.

Choose a decaffeinated variety of tea if caffeine is a problem for you. You can also make a caffeine-free tea substitute by steeping some fresh or dried culinary herbs and spices in hot water. You can put them in a cloth bag, but I put them in loose in order to chew and eat them, after or as I sip the tea.

Herbal tea can be made of the parts of many plants: flowers, berries, roots, seeds, and bark.

Basic Tea Preparation

Allow 1 teaspoon to 1 tablespoon of tea for 1 cup of water. For all tea, use filtered water. If you don't have it, then prepare tap water by letting it sit overnight in a glass container so the chlorine will evaporate. The water for black tea should be boiling, but for green tea, which is more delicate, let the boiling water sit for five minutes before using.

Pour the water over your tea. Cover, and let the tea steep for 2 to 5 minutes. Use this strong brew as a base and fill one third of your cup with the base, then fill with plain hot water before drinking. Before serving, remember to make sure that your tea is not too hot. For iced tea, mix the base with cold water and add ice. But it is best to drink it warm, after a meal. Seal and refrigerate the leftover base to use the next day.

Many women find that ginseng in their morning tea gives them a pleasant sense of alertness without the jittery feeling of caffeine. The tropical hibiscus flower makes a wonderful addition of antioxidant to tea, adding a tart, refreshing taste. It may have a mild laxative and diuretic effect. Rooibos (pronounced rue-buys), or red tea, from an African plant, has no caffeine or tannic acid and is a powerful antioxidant.

SERVING TEA

Cultural wisdom suggests, when drinking tea, to take a deep breath and be aware of your own presence. Enjoy the fragrance and presence of the tea. Hold the cup in both hands and savor the feel of its warmth or its coolness before you take a sip of your tea. Sniff the aroma and chew a leaf or two to experience the flavor sensation in different areas of your mouth.

You can heighten flavor by sweetening your tea with some raisins or dates, or small hard ginger or natural licorice candies, or jazz it up with a little honey, spices, fruit, and almond, soy, or rice milk. In fact, additions to tea are an important technique in most tea-drinking cultures.

Women of the Ukraine gather berries and fruit to make jam, which can be stored, and then stir this jam into hot water to make tea.

Teatime can be fun—make it a special occasion by sharing a cup with family and friends. Or, don't stand on ritual and ceremony just drink tea to your health.

TEATIME MEDITATION

Even if you already know what meditation is all about and have your own program for relaxation and self-awareness, your mind can still open wider, and your well-being can still be heightened. Meditation is associated with mindfulness-breathing techniques and with tea-drinking cultures.

How does one begin to meditate—to, in the beginning, find time? Some say, read a poem. Have you ever meditated upon the meanings in poetry as a way to find meaning in your own life? That music can enhance meditation and relaxation is well-known in all cultures.

You can combine tea and meditation in one or more ways. Here are some suggestions:

- Take a meditation walk or do a qigong warm-up, then refresh yourself with tea.

- Write about your life in your journal between tea snacks.

- Read a little about another country to transport yourself.

- Share poems of thoughts from faraway places or cultural wisdom.

- Read a poem from a poet you enjoy.

- Welcome a guest and serve tea. ❧

cultural wisdom about every breath you take

Many ancient spiritual and physical practices incorporate breathing exercises. Yoga combines *prana* or *pranayama* (moving life force or breath) with *asanas*, or postures. The union of the physical and spiritual culminates in meditation, which is the reason to achieve physical stamina and flexibility and breath control. *Qigong*, brought to the West from China, uses breath to move the *qi*, or life force, energy throughout the body. Movements are designed to move breath and energy into certain organs and along meridians, healing and toning. Ayurvedic health practices include cleansing breaths.

Breathing has been used as part of psychotherapy in the West because practitioners believe breath has the power to reach into the subconscious and heal emotional trauma (Ley 1999). It has also been used to enhance healing from cancer and other life-threatening diseases (Manon et al. 2003). You can use breath in stressful situations to calm and nurture yourself.

Breath and life force remain woven together in most cultural traditions, and Western women are awakening to the power of this natural process. Breathing consciously should be part of each day, and finding time to practice the breathing exercises later in this chapter will reward any health or movement program you follow. Combine conscious breathing with an appreciation of the atmosphere around you, welcoming the freshness of spring or the astringent fall air as you awaken to the beauty of nature and your body's power to heal.

COMBINING BREATHING & MOVEMENT

Movement stimulates our muscles, organs, cells, neurotransmitters, and hormones and keeps us youthful. Stretching, weight lifting, walking, running, dancing, or practicing qigong: each builds strength, stamina, and flexibility and keeps our muscles doing what they were meant to do. Movement practices are designed to increase our respiration and heart rate, and serve to strengthen our cardiovascular and muscular systems. You can use exercise to increase brain power, elevate moods, increase sex drive, keep flexible, and stimulate your organs to heal. Meditation and visualization begin with concentrating on our own breathing cycles, lengthening and deepening the breath, bringing the life-force energy into each cell.

Breathing and movement, for most of us, are automatic functions. We do not think about breathing, yet it happens continuously for each of us. Movement, although more conscious, does not require the same thought as, say, choosing a job or driving a car. Yet by consciously participating in breathing and movements, you can increase your health awareness and create a strong communication between your body and mind.

INHALE LIFE & EXHALE TO LET GO

Breath is intricately connected to our emotional lives. As we relax, our breaths get longer and deeper. If we feel anger, our breathing speeds up and becomes shallower, sometimes with panting exhalations. Deep sorrow causes us to breathe spasmodically, with superficial, uneven breaths, much like sobbing. Guilt or anxiety can make us feel we are being suffocated, as though we are no longer taking in life. Feelings of love or contentment soften our breath and smooth it. By sitting or standing beside someone experiencing anger or anxiety and breathing slowly and calmly, you can alter the person's breathing and help them reach a state of calmness. Often, the fatigue associated with depression or getting older is a direct result of lack of oxygen. I remember my mother handling stress and depression by taking walks. Whenever she felt these symptoms coming on, she would stop whatever she was doing and go out into the fresh air for a brisk stroll. She would inevitably return refreshed, with a better mood and renewed energy. Now I practice walking for stress relief. Breath is a powerful tool for both physical and emotional well-being.

Our lungs are expanding bellows reaching from our collarbones to our abdomen. Using this entire lung capacity may be a new experience for you. Take a minute right now to test this statement: Stand as straight as possible wherever you are. Breathe a few normal breaths, and then place your hands lightly on your abdomen. Exhale through your nose, feeling the diaphragm muscle move inward as it pushes out the air. Inhale, feeling the diaphragm move outward naturally. Take as deep a breath as possible. Next, hook your thumbs into your armpits and rest your palms and fingers lightly on your upper chest. Breath out and in again, feeling the expansion in your chest this time.

The capacity of the lungs is huge, and the more oxygen you take in with breath, the more energy is available to each cell. Conversely, the more toxins you can expel with each exhalation, the cleaner your body becomes. By consciously using the full capacity of your lungs, you can improve your capacity for taking in oxygen. The following breathing exercises should help you increase your lung capacity while nourishing your body, invigorating your spirit, and calming your mind.

Breath of Life

The following breathing exercise takes no more than fifteen minutes but will have a tremendous positive impact. Try it a few times, and you'll see what I mean. This practice incorporates oxygen, sunlight, and tea—crucial foods for every woman.

Prepare your morning tea. Choose a quiet place to sit, if possible by a window where you can look out toward the morning light. If you can, open the window to feel the fresh morning breeze.

Breathe life in deeply through the aroma of your tea, gaze at the color of the liquid, and feel the steam rise to your cheek. Close your eyes and hold the warm cup between your hands as the warmth infuses your body. Let the fragrance envelope you—the heady scents of peppermint, lemon leaves, orange peel, or ginger. Breathe in fresh energy from the morning, and, as you let go of each breath, let go of tension or concerns.

If you like, visualize yourself in a pine forest, in a flower garden, on a wave-cleansed beach, or floating freely through the blue sky as a bird. Feel the wisps of mist and the warmth of the sun. Imagine you are breathing in that air.

Now, come to your own place on earth. Rub your hands together to create warmth, then immediately place one palm over each eye as you breathe in and breathe out.

Gently massage both eyelids with your palms. When you feel comfortable, remove your hands and open your eyes slowly. You have given your body and mind a relaxation exercise.

Breathing for Healthy Lungs

To clear the lungs and build stamina, sit or stand in a comfortable position. Place your tongue lightly on the roof of your mouth just behind your front teeth. Breathe in for four counts through your nose. Hold the air for five counts, and then exhale through your mouth for ten counts. Do this for several cycles, and then return to normal breathing.

Once you've practiced a few times, increase the time you inhale to eight counts, hold for eight, and exhale for sixteen. The goal is to exhale for twice as long as you inhale. This exercise is effective at getting rid of stress and centering yourself, especially if you often feel out of breath or short of breath. You can practice it while walking, for example, to help control your breath. The longer you exhale, the more room there is in your lungs for fresh air and the more you let go of what you don't need.

Herbs that help lungs are clover, lemon balm, milk thistle, and lavender. Try them in your tea. Scents for aromatherapy for the lungs are clove, cinnamon, melissa, and lavender.

Breathing for Concentration, Energy, & to Massage Organs

You can do this exercise with your eyes closed or open, but focus inward.

Let your stomach be soft as you breathe in through your nostrils, slowly. Feel your diaphragm expand downward as your lungs fill with air. Expand your stomach out, but don't expand your chest. Hold the breath gently for a moment and then exhale it through your mouth, letting your stomach collapse inward as your lungs empty and as your diaphragm gently pushes the air out. As you practice this, try to exhale for a longer time than you inhale. After you are able to do this easily, add this next part of the exercise: Once the air is in your stomach, move it up into your chest by constricting your stomach. Do not exhale but lock your chin and move the air, holding it for a count of three, then exhaling. This will massage your internal organs.

Breathing Exercise for the Gastrointestinal Tract

This is a relaxing breathing exercise that has proven effective for women with digestive problems. The action of breathing helps to move the fluids of your lymphatic system through your body. The lymphatic system moves large particles from the intestines and other organs into the bloodstream and helps to keep the fingerlike protrusions (villi) of the intestines drained.

Sit with your feet flat on the floor and your spine straight. Close your eyes gently and breathe in and out to relax. Bring your palms together in front of your face and rub them vigorously together. This warms them and activates your body's internal healing mechanisms. Place your hands lightly on your knees, palms on top and fingers resting on the three notches of your knee. If you place your hands in this position, you will feel the notches I mean. Bring your attention to your breath, feeling your belly move in and out with each breath. Don't change your breathing, simply observe it and hold the notches firmly with your fingers. Keep your mind focused on the movement of your belly with each breath. Do this for several minutes, and your digestive organs will relax and move around, massaging each other. The lymph system will flow smoothly, and you may experience better digestion.

Breathing Exercise for Nerves & Hormones

Use this wonderful exercise for calming your nerves or for going to sleep at night. You can use it to overcome insomnia, along with a snack of carbohydrates and noncaffeinated tea. Sit or lie comfortably, with your clothes loose around your waist to allow your diaphragm to expand fully. Rest your hands, palms down, lightly on your thighs. If you are lying down, rest your arms beside you, palms up.

Lengthen your spine and make it as straight as possible, thinking of a pulley or a balloon lifting the crown of your head. Relax your shoulders. One good way to do this if you are standing or sitting, is to raise your shoulders to your ears and then release them, pushing them down and back. Take a few normal breaths through your nostrils, allowing the air to expand and fill your lungs. Breathe in through your nose as you count to four, allowing your abdomen to expand as you draw air deep into your lungs. Hold it softly there while counting to four. Breathe out through your nose for four counts, allowing your diaphragm muscle to gently push all the air out of your lungs. Count to four with no air in your lungs. Begin again by breathing in through your nose for four counts, holding the air for four counts, breathing out for four counts, and holding no air for four counts. After you have practiced this exercise a few times, lengthen each count to six counts, then eight counts. If you feel light-headed while practicing, simply stop for a few moments and breathe normally, then resume. ❧

move through your life for fitness & fun

Our bodies were built to move, and move gracefully, just as birds were built to soar through the sky and cats were made to stretch and leap. Make your daily movements a celebration of the strength, grace, and flexibility of your body. Take an energetic walk somewhere beautiful. Lift weights to your favorite music. Take someone you love to a dancing class. Play tennis or basketball with someone you'd like to spend more time with. Choose a variety of activities, and do them with other people as often as possible. Make movement fun by whistling and singing as you walk. Let the music come from inside, not from a recording you carry. Experiment with sounds. Hum a tune, or whistle. Greet strangers with a musical hello.

Variety—in movement and activities, as in food—is better than too much of any one thing. I am practicing and studying qigong but find walking is the best time to think. My friend Karen found that aerobic exercise did not work for her when she was recovering from cancer treatments and she now practices qigong and tai chi. The important thing is to include some movement each day, and to set a goal of spending at least three hours each week in movement—about thirty minutes six times a week, or fifteen minutes twice each day.

Exercise increases endorphins for elevated moods, balances insulin for steady blood sugar through the day, increases the body's ability to eliminate toxins, and raises your metabolism to burn more calories and provide energy. And you don't need to become a marathon runner to improve your overall physical fitness or receive the benefits. Researchers at Johns Hopkins University determined that adding more physical activity in any form—walking, gardening, or engaging in everyday activities—will improve lung and heart capacity (Infeld et al. 1997). Exercise does not have to be incredibly vigorous or uninterrupted. Participants in the study were able to improve their stamina, increase muscle tone, and lose weight with walking and other low-impact activities. Getting in shape does not mean you need to go to a gym or invest in equipment. The goal is to become more active.

CULTURAL TRADITIONS OF EVERYDAY MOVEMENT

In many areas around the world, women do not think about exercising but simply do it as part of their everyday activities. For example, in Asia, gasoline is expensive and most people don't own cars. Women in Vietnam and China bicycle or walk everywhere, to market and back, to social gatherings, or to jobs. In rural areas of Hungary and for Bedouin tribes of Morocco and the Sinai, horses are basic transport. In many areas of Europe, cars are not allowed on village streets and people walk, carrying baskets for groceries and other purchases. Greece and Italy are a maze of narrow pathways, too narrow for cars but perfect for walking. As they walk these paths, women are rewarded with glimpses of the beautiful azure sea, ancient white stones, and bright sky.

Fitness and exercise should be part of your everyday life, too. You can walk the extra blocks to the post office rather than jumping in your car, or take the stairs instead of the elevator in your office building. Gardening provides exercise while connecting you to nature, and perhaps helping you eat better with fresh vegetables and herbs. Mowing the lawn, shoveling snow, energetic scrubbing, all of these provide exercise. Each time you have a chore, think how you can incorporate movement or breathing.

Exercise improves moods by balancing neurotransmitters and releasing endorphins, increases self-esteem, releases stress, helps you lose fat and gain muscle, improves skin, aids regularity and digestion, strengthens bones, prevents heart disease, increases metabolism, helps you sleep restfully, and may lengthen your life. It increases muscle mass for a toned and beautiful body. Exercise balances insulin and other hormonal activity and balances electrolytes to prevent bloating and other digestive problems. Your fitness and movement should include stretching for flexibility (such as yoga) weight-bearing for strong bones and to prevent osteoporosis, and aerobic exercise and deep breathing for circulation and heart strengthening. Many types of exercise incorporate one or more of these.

In addition, qigong, yoga, tai chi, and other movement practices improve circulation, flexibility, and stamina as well as boost your respiratory system.

ARE YOU AN ATHLETE?

Moderate exercise should be part of every woman's life, but some women enjoy the challenge of sports and physical exertion and push themselves to ever higher levels of fitness. Athletic women of all ages should make sure that they are getting all the nutrients and non-nutrients they need and that they are replenishing their bodies with rest after strenuous activity. Essential fatty acids are important for joint lubrication, and nuts and seeds are good sources. Contrary to popular belief, meat and animal products are not necessary to maintain high levels of physical exertion.

Just as too much of any one food is not good for you, too much exercise can be unhealthy. Some athletic women avoid eating any type of fat and train so strenuously that they stop menstruating and experience other unhealthy consequences. Athletes need to include essential fatty acids and other crucial foods in their diets to maintain a healthy percentage of body fat and hormone balance. Strenuous exercise can cause food cravings in some women. If you are athletic, be sure to eat foods high in chromium, such as olives, grapes, peanuts, whole grains, kelp, alfalfa, or broccoli. These foods will help eliminate cravings. Inability to lose weight even with increased physical exercise may be due to an underlying food sensitivity. Because women's knees are more vulnerable to injury than men's, you should avoid doing leg extensions, deep knee bends, or any other activity that causes knee pain or extreme knee stress.

FOOD WISDOM MOVEMENT GOALS

You can use your food diary to set some new movement goals. As you accomplish them, set new ones. Here are some examples:

- *"One day this week, I will get up fifteen minutes early to practice Breath of Life breathing or meditation."*

- *"I will take a walk alone during my break twice this week and practice a walking mediation."*

- *"In the evening, I will ask my friend, husband, neighbor, or child to take a walk with me in a park nearby."*

- *"Three times this week, I will find the time to move—walk, dance, play tennis, run, or practice qigong—for at least thirty minutes."*

- *"I will learn a dance step, and practice it to music."*

- *"Three times each day—morning, before dinner, and before bed—I will practice conscious breathing for five minutes."*

After choosing three goals for this week, choose three long-term goals for the month, practices that you will continue on a daily or weekly basis for one month. Get out with your artistic self and move—breathing as you go. For more on breathing exercises, see www.drsonia.com.

chapter 6

snacking your way to good health

A lover's food is the love of bread,
Not the bread.
—Rumi

snacks are our moments of refreshment delight. When
we reach for a snack we often feel a rush of pleasure. Even if our snack
lasts only ten or twenty minutes, we look forward to it and enjoy it. The
food wisdom snacking way will help you create your own take-out
kitchen with food on the move that replenishes your cells, brain, and
hormones while satisfying your snacking urges.

Snacks can be portable, succulent morsels of health and power-
houses of nutrients. To make it easy to eat little bits of ecstasy, your
healthful snack food can be packaged in its own rind, skin, or shell: a
plum, a kiwi, a cucumber, a handful of almonds. Or you can put together
a formula once a week in your own kitchen (see recipes in this chapter
and in chapter 10), and divide it neatly into baggies that you can take
anywhere.

wise snacking

I can't say enough about the importance of snacking on your most important nutrients, oxygen and water!

Water is on the topmost level of the food pyramid and, as an alternative to less-healthy snacking, is good for many reasons. One good reason for carrying water and taking frequent sips is that you can think more clearly, as water has almost immediate action in the brain.

Lucy came to me with problems of anxiety and exhaustion and said she felt the need to eat "all day." Her normal day started very early and she drove from meeting to meeting throughout the congested San Francisco area. I suggested she drink tea or plain water a half hour before eating solid food and when she became hungry to drink first. I also told her to take slow deep breaths every time she felt hungry—three deep breaths with her eyes closed (except when she was driving). Taking the time to replenish her oxygen supply and rest her mind briefly gave her more energy than a candy bar or food. Try snacking on tea, water, and air, and seeing how invigorating it can be. ❧

learn to snack
on healthy food

If you were raised not to eat between meals, because "it spoils your appetite" or because "snacking makes you fat," you can appreciate and admire your independent spirit, your little rebellion, if you are a frequent snacker. Wanting to snack on a salty or sugary food is a learned habit, just as with any other food choices, and it's a habit you can break.

To begin, use your food diary to keep track of all the foods you eat, paying particular attention this week to your snacks between meals. Take a few minutes to respond to these questions:

- *How many times do you eat each day, counting snacks?*

- *Do you crave sweets? Salty foods? Starchy foods? Crunchy foods? Fatty foods? Other types of food? What time of day do you usually experience cravings?*

- *Do you often feel hungry between meals or all the time but avoid eating for fear of gaining weight? Does this happen at a particular time each day, such as midmorning, midafternoon, or before bedtime?*

- *Are there times throughout the day that you feel low energy? Do you eat in response to this lull?*

- *Do you snack when you get bored?*

- *Do you usually choose snacks that are convenient? Inexpensive? Purchased in advance? Purchased from vending machines?*

- *Do you carry any foods with you daily?*

- *Do you ever carry snack foods with you when you travel? When you're in the car?*

- *Can you name the cause of your undesired snacking habits, if any, as emotional or physical hunger?* ❧

the american way of snacking

The way we have learned to snack in our culture tells us something about the health of our society. Snacks are available everywhere we turn, and in a dizzying array of varieties; there is no other food group that receives so much media promotion.

Many of the most popular snacks in Western cultures include excess fat, salt, starch, sugar, or caffeine. Most manufactured snacks contain artificial substances which may cause problems, such as interference with your blood sugar, or encouraging cravings and weight imbalance. Commercial food companies have gradually led Americans to feel that our snacks should be packaged foods, often with chemically developed sweeteners or fats. Some commercial snacks cause headaches and fatigue, contribute to tooth decay, and may increase anxiety and mood swings.

I cannot pass judgment on laboratory-developed or factory-processed snacks, as we have not lived with them for centuries to know how they serve our health over time. What I am saying is that fiber, whole plant foods, antioxidants, herbs, spices, essential fatty acids, and quality protein are needed to maintain wellness. We live in a fast-paced world, with products continually vying for our attention and with new research results constantly in the news. But, ultimately no one cares about your well-being more than you do, and you must discover for yourself what foods work best for you. ❧

the positive value of snacking

Snacking is a quick way to get food and energy. The quick energy from snacking can help you perform better, and snacks are easy to fix when you don't have time to cook. They can be economical. Some of my clients find healthy snacking keeps their weight and blood sugar stable, balances mood, and helps relieve other symptoms. Snacking can also help you get the nutrients and fiber you need if you know you didn't get the right food during a regular meal. You may use snacks to prevent symptoms such as headaches, shakiness, or fatigue. Or you may snack simply because you enjoy it. ❧

snacking to satisfy your basic urges

It is especially important to be attentive as to why you are choosing certain foods for snacks. Two basic urges that are sometimes confused by the brain are emotional and physical hunger. Your choices might be based on flavor or on subliminal memories of feeling good or bad. By using your food diary, you'll discover the reasons you snack and what foods bring satisfaction and provide longer-lasting energy. As with all food choices, successful snacking requires building the right habits.

You can change your habits gradually, perhaps once a day or a few times each week at first, and let your body absorb the benefits. As your blood chemistry balances and your body feel more harmonious, it will be easier to choose healthy snacks more often and to eliminate some of the foods that don't provide nutrition. A first step to breaking old habits might be to use tea to occupy your mind and mouth rather than eating something. You'll learn to distinguish between hunger and thirst, because often sipping tea for hydration and oral pleasure will be what your body needs more than solid food. ❧

eat low glycemic foods for steady energy

Your energy level depends, in part, on the amount of blood sugar you have, which in turn depends on your insulin level. Carbohydrates have been rated according to their *glycemic index*, a measure of the rate at which they are broken down into glucose and released into the blood. A high glycemic index means that sugar or starch will quickly raise your blood sugar. Protein, fiber, and fat slow a food's breakdown, while processing speeds it up. Snacking on high-sugar foods will spike your blood sugar, giving you a quick lift and then a quick fall into tiredness. On the other hand, snacking throughout the day on medium or low glycemic foods such as complex carbohydrates, especially combined with plant proteins (apple or celery with ricotta cheese) and other plant foods, can help you maintain your energy. Balancing levels of insulin and blood sugar with foods with a low glycemic index may help you prevent cravings or impulsive eating.

TIFFANY'S STORY

Tiffany first came to me complaining of low energy, PMS, and severe pain during her periods. She was in her late twenties and had always been physically active, especially as a dance major in college. After college, however, she took an office job and found herself becoming less and less active. She had gotten into the habit of boosting her energy before dance classes with candy bars and diet soft drinks with caffeine. She had recently started taking birth control pills and was gaining weight. She took multivitamins and other supplements to counteract the fatigue. Tiffany had tried various diets unsuccessfully. When she came to me, I suggested she snack on foods that provide long-term energy, such as an apple with almond butter or sliced tomatoes with hummus. She became interested in reading labels, looking for snacks with no artificial ingredients. She discovered that certain wasabi chips, potato chips, and other vegetable chips had 6 grams of fat and 130 calories per half cup. She sometimes used these for snacking, and to compensate for the higher calories she decided to do twenty minutes of extra exercise. Tiffany continued taking multivitamins, but I added enzymes, vitamin E, extra B complex and B_6, and suggested more foods high in chromium (mushrooms, whole grains, and asparagus).

"Eventually, my new snacking habits did for me what the other foods couldn't," Tiffany said later. "My thyroid measurement and progesterone balance became normal within four months. My last three periods have been so peaceful—no PMS, very few cravings, no pain—that I'm surprised that I'm having my period. I no longer have bloating or pain in my stomach and gas in my bowels. Best of all, I don't carry bags of junk food around anymore; instead I am carrying healthy snacks. Now, I look forward to challenges and new experiences because I feel good and I feel in control. My hair is back to its previous shining and manageable full state, too. Now, instead of sleeping all weekend, I go skiing."

Tiffany had never been aware of the types of food she was depending on for fuel, and noting these snacks in her food diary each day allowed her to recognize what she ate. Slowly, she realized that these foods, even though many of them had been her favorites for many years, were not providing her with what she needed. She could see this because she was recording her symptoms in her daily food diary; as a result she was able to slowly change to healthy foods and build new associations with these foods.

Pick-Me-Up Tea

½ cup green tea
½ cup dandelion greens or spearmint
2 tablespoons each cardamom and
   chopped licorice root

Follow the basic tea preparation method (see chapter 5). Serve with figs, butter toffee, peanuts, or ginger candy.

Many snacking habits are learned in childhood. You may associate a sense of belonging and happiness with these foods. If they give you emotional comfort, just use them less frequently and begin building new food habits, ones based on aromas and flavors that feed your spirit and your body. Associate your new food choices with fun, love, companionship, and a happy experience. Taste and smell are more closely associated with pleasure or displeasure than the senses of sight or sound. ❧

mother nature's bountiful plant foods

I want you to think of every imaginable edible whole plant food as a convenient, tasty treat to enjoy snacking on: as simple, easy-to-prepare, easy-to-carry, and easy-to-digest protein, with protective antioxidants, phytonutrients, minerals, and essential fatty acids. Fruits, vegetables, and roasted grains and beans make excellent snacks. Here are some healthy snack ideas.

Tiffany inspired me to create a new bag of snacks, a bag of healthy snacks that my clients and others carry with them all the time. This snack can contain whatever you like best or whatever you happen to buy in a given week, including ingredients you haven't used before. When you get a craving for a snack, grab a handful of whatever is in your bag, and feed your body, mind, and cells. ❧

Roasted Garbanzos or Soybeans

MAKES 3 CUPS ROASTED BEANS
   2 cups garbanzo beans or soybeans
   4 cups water, at room temperature
   Pinch of salt, cayenne, lemon, cumin, cinnamon, or honey, to taste

Rinse the beans in a colander and pick out any stones or dirt. Add the beans to a bowl with the water, and soak for ten to twelve hours.
Drain the beans and spread them on a cookie sheet or other flat baking pan.
Preheat the oven to 350°F.
Sprinkle with your choice of the spices and flavorings listed.
Bake for 1 hour, checking for desired crunchiness.

Variation: *For wheat berries and lentils follow the same directions, except reduce soaking time by half. Amaranth and buckwheat don't need any soaking; place them dry on a pan in a 350° F oven for 20 to 25 minutes to roast or puff, or 3 to 5 minutes per cup in a microwave.*

Snack on these roasted legumes plain, or add them to your salad.

indulge your senses with healthy choices

Regardless of what is good for us, foods need to have flavor. Therefore, I've put together snacks with flavor in mind, but these snacks also provide balanced acidic-alkaline qualities, phytohormonals, antioxidants, and fiber. All of these snacks can be taken along with you or fixed quickly at home any time of the day. Many can be expanded to create balanced meals, too. I've divided them into two lists here, for your convenience.

Boshki's Travel Snack

Use ½ to 2 cups of any or all of the following: pumpkin seeds, almonds (slivered or whole), peanuts, sesame seeds, roasted garbanzo beans, roasted soybeans, dried prunes, flaxseeds, pecans, candied ginger, dried papaya, raisins, dried figs, dates, walnuts, granola, and roasted rice or other grains. (For roasted garbanzos, soybeans, and grains, see preceding recipe.)

Mix everything together. All of these ingredients will stay fresh for weeks without refrigeration. If you tend eat a lot of chocolate candy, try adding small amounts of M&Ms or other such treats into this if you desire. You'll eat less of the candy, but still enjoy the taste.

High-protein snacks: Boshki's Travel Snack; sardines or tuna on a cracker; yogurt with fruit and nuts; veggie burger; hummus dip with vegetables and greens; falafel with tahini sauce or pomegranate sauce; roasted, dried, or canned garbanzos, lentils, or soybeans; cereal with milk or yogurt, fruits, and nuts or seeds; barbecued tofu; ricotta or feta spread on toast, or mixed with fruit and herbs; tuna with lemon and parsley and bread; hard-boiled eggs; ricotta or cottage cheese with melon and pumpkin seeds; potato filled with ricotta cheese; half a turkey or cheese sandwich; green salad with hard-boiled egg white or feta cheese with sesame seeds and olive oil.

High-fiber snacks: dried or fresh fruits; raw vegetables; baked potato with green onions (or chives) and olives; canned bean soup with whole wheat crackers; roasted beans; cooked root vegetables; marinated sliced ginger or other pickled

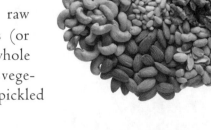

vegetables; fresh sliced or pickled seaweed; sushi seaweed wrap; gazpacho; greens and herbs; sliced mango, fresh mint leaves, and chopped walnuts on a brown rice cake; Calming Persian Cold Yogurt Soup (see chapter 10); lettuce with mushrooms, olives, and feta cheese; spring rolls; rice cakes or crackers; corn muffin with oranges or orange marmalade; English muffin with almond butter or jam; Silky Fruity Muffins (see chapter 4) and Tea for Life (see chapter 5); raisin bread toast with ginger or ginseng tea; cereal eaten like chips; seeds.

INDULGE YOUR SWEET TOOTH—HEALTHFULLY!

By following the food wisdom pyramid and eating five to six small meals a day, with a variety of carbohydrates, proteins, essential fatty acids, fiber, and phytonutrients right from your first snack or meal, you can prevent a craving for sweets. And, if you do have a craving, eating whole foods that offer sweetness will provide your body with real fuel. If you feel low energy before or after working out, for example, you might want to try some complex carbohydrate or protein snacks. These can enhance your performance.

One of the first things the women I counsel usually experience when they add more whole plant food into their diets is that they lose their craving for sweets. Such cravings are a familiar side effect of unbalanced insulin and estrogen for many women, and especially for menopausal women and women with PMS. Estrogen stimulates the brain cells that produce serotonin and influences the secretions from the thyroid and pancreas. Simple sugars will increase blood sugar quickly, causing a sharp decline after a sharp increase in energy. When you eat complex carbohydrates, which are generally high in fiber and phytohormones, your brain produces the right amount of serotonin. When brain serotonin levels are normal, you feel satisfied and calm. When serotonin is too low, you crave sweets since they're the quickest way to get carbohydrates.

If you are eating nutritionally most of the time, having a fudge brownie, donut, or cookies once in a while will not do much harm. But snacks such as pumpkin seeds, seaweed, cereal with yogurt or soy milk, figs, nuts, vegetables, and legumes have a beneficial effect on serotonin levels. Rather than worry about how many sweet foods to eat, let your body say when enough is enough. If you are watching your weight, a quarter cup of dried fruit or two to three slices of melon, ginger candies, or ginger snaps is a good place to start.

Snacks for a sweets craving: dried fruits, chewy and sweet but packed with fiber, such as apricots, cherries, raisins, or apples; dried or fresh berries; tea with an almond biscotti or a cookie; crystallized ginger with nuts; ginger candies; ginger snaps; melon; chai latte with almond or soy milk. ❧

snack foods & fat

Too much hydrogenated fat and trans-fatty acids in our diets may inhibit the absorption of essential fatty acids—the good fats—and cause cell damage. As a home chef and nutritionist I always choose cold-pressed virgin olive oil, as it is the oil closest to nature and the oil which keeps flavor best. Other choices are grape seed oil, sesame oil, and walnut oil. You can use less oil and still enjoy the flavor. Milder oil does not satisfy as well when you have a strong desire for taste and flavor. If you want butter because it satisfies, eat extra fiber food to take the fat out of your system better, and do extra exercise to use up the calories.

Hydrogenated fats, sometimes called trans-fatty acids, are fats created by a chemical process in which hydrogen is added to naturally occurring polyunsaturated fats. Hydrogenated fats are stable and have long shelf lives, making them desirable to food companies, but inhibit the body's ability to absorb naturally occurring fatty acids and other nutrients. Margarine, cookies, cakes, and other prepackaged foods contain trans-fatty acids. These fats may be more harmful in causing cancer than other fats. Hydrogenated fats also may be related to heart disease.

PORTABLE POWERHOUSES: SNACKING FOR ANTIOXIDANTS & ESSENTIAL FATTY ACIDS

Snacking on seeds and nuts gives you a good source of vitamin E and its antioxidant functions in the body. Vitamin E is especially important for maintaining cell membranes in red blood cells. It can help to prevent damage caused by air pollution and environmental toxins. Nuts and seeds are also convenient packages of nutrients and phytonutrients, including essential fatty acids, protein, phytohormones, antioxidants, and fiber. The body does not manufacture essential fatty acids; eating snacks that contain small quantities of these elements is crucial to your health.

The need for vitamin E decreases if you are receiving selenium through whole grains and other foods, but snacking on rich sources of this essential antioxidant is a good idea. Sources include flaxseeds, sunflower seeds, pumpkin seeds, olives, wheat germ, whole grains, walnuts, and almonds.

You can choose one to two snacks a day from the following list to meet your good-fat needs; these snacks are also high in fiber.

Essential fatty acid snacks: flaxseeds mixed with flavorful sesame seeds; French olives, Greek olives, green or black olives; plate of hummus and olives; bread dipped in garlic-flavored olive oil or spread with tapenade; avocado, sesame seeds, basil or mint, and tomato wrapped in seaweed sheets (available in many ethnic markets); guacamole with pita chips; walnut butter, cashew butter, sesame butter, or peanut butter spread on apples, celery, or crackers; sardines on crackers; nut sauce, flaxseed oil, or garlic-flavored olive oil on kale, bok choy, or spinach. 🍃

Essential All-Health-Purpose Hummus

MAKES 4 TO 6 SERVINGS

Use this recipe for a filling to stuff into pita bread pockets and take it along to snack on as needed. Women in the Mediterranean have eaten hummus as a snack or served it as a main course for generations. Hummus is great for children, to help them build strong bones, and for menopausal women, who need to keep their bones strong. You can eat this treat over several days. The flavor improves if you make it a day ahead. Serve hummus with toasted pita bread or crackers and arugula, olives, and tomatoes, and garnish with mint, olive oil, and cayenne pepper.

> **2½ cups cooked or canned garbanzos, drained**
> **1 cup soft tofu (about 5 ounces), drained (optional)**
> **½ cup tahini or ground sesame seeds**
> **½ cup flaxseeds or ground black sesame seeds**
> **1 tablespoon olive oil**
> **¼ cup fresh lemon juice**
> **½ cup each chopped fresh parsley and chopped tomato (optional)**
> **½ medium red onion, diced**
> **3 cloves fresh garlic**
> **1 teaspoon cayenne or to taste**
> **Salt and black pepper to taste**

Combine all the ingredients except salt and pepper in a food processor and puree until smooth. Season to taste with salt and pepper.

snacks for specific body systems

For more snack ideas, try the recipes in chapter 10, or try one of the following.

High-energy quick snack: Use roasted soy, garbanzo, dried lentil or black bean flakes, and raisins bought in bulk in natural food stores as a flavorful, low-fat high-energy snack.

Easy digestion snacks: Snack on cardamom seeds to aid digestion: crack the soft pod with your teeth and eat the tiny, pungent seeds inside. They have a strong, pleasant taste and will freshen your breath. Chewing fresh parsley will aid digestion, prevent bloating, and balance hormones, reducing discomfort during PMS and perimenopause. Parsley freshens your breath and stimulates your taste buds.

Assorted snacks for hot-cold balance: If you are feeling cold, try some ginger candy with roasted nuts and cinnamon. If you are feeling hot, try a slice of watermelon, or chew on cilantro, mint, dill seeds, prunes, or cucumber-yogurt salad sprinkled with fresh dill.

Easy energy snack: Need to prepare for a meeting? Eat a handful of almonds. Feeling low energy? Try some roasted garbanzos or soybeans. Another easy idea: just keep a container of fresh yogurt in the refrigerator at work or at home and carry a few vegetables to eat each day. Top with fresh herbs or seeds from your seed bag, and you have a complete, balanced approach to an afternoon snack.

Women's flavorful watercress calcium snack: Women should become familiar with watercress, a flavorful green and herb believed to contribute to longevity in many cultures. Watercress is high in calcium and iodine and may help balance thyroid function and metabolism and treat yeast overgrowth. Add it to salads and sandwiches, or simply nibble it with any meal. ❧

more snacking way

Here are a few more tasty alternatives.

- Pickled snacks: One great way to preserve foods, used for centuries, is by pickling. I keep a jar in my refrigerator at all times with fresh vegetables being pickled. Unpeeled garlic cloves, sliced or thick-cut chunks of Jerusalem artichoke, sliced cabbage, and onions combine well with dill weed, fenugreek, and vinegar. Fill the jar and cover the vegetables, spices, and herbs with apple cider vinegar. The fenugreek aids digestion and the vinegar will help balance your body's acidity and alkalinity. The flavor is enhanced over time, and the foods retain all their vital nutrients, phytochemicals, and fibers. They provide bursts of flavor and a satisfying crunchiness.

- Roasting seeds and spices (such as cumin): Toss seeds into a dry skillet over medium heat for three to five minutes, or until they are fragrant and a little browned, stirring as they get hot. They should brown slightly without sticking. An alternative is to put a handful on a square of aluminum foil or in a small ovenproof pan and place under the broiler for five minutes. Take care not to burn them. The heat brings out the flavors, but use them immediately after roasting so that the oils do not turn rancid. These make a great snack as well as a garnish.

- Crunchy snacks: Cucumbers satisfy our desire for crunchy foods and hydrate and cool us. Keep a bag of small cucumbers in your car or purse. They'll keep for several days without refrigeration, and they make a quick refreshing snack as you run errands. The French, Dutch, and other Europeans enjoy sliced radish with salt and pepper on crusty bread for breakfast or as a snack with their tea. Snacks in Mexico include raw jicama sliced and sprinkled with paprika or lemon juice. In Hungary, a slice of red or yellow bell pepper with a hard-boiled egg or a square inch of cheese can be breakfast or a snack. ❧

snacks not listed

I haven't included any of the snacks of choice for many Americans, such as ice cream, candy bars, potato chips, energy bars, or chocolate, all of which are loaded with sugar or fat. If you eat these occasionally, don't stop eating them entirely unless you feel like it; eating them now and then will not harm your overall good health, and breaking the habit cold turkey will probably be too difficult. When you do eat them, include a healthy fruit creatively, the way Melanie, a cute little nine-year-old, has learned to do. She recently served me strawberries she had dipped in chocolate by herself. Holding the tray of these fruits with their pretty green stems and half of the juicy red berry showing above the chocolate, she said, "My daddy is a chocoholic, so when I make these he doesn't get too much, because too much is too much." Such a wise little girl.

BALANCE YOUR SODIUM INTAKE

The body needs sodium, which is an electrolyte that aids internal chemical reactions, but an imbalance of sodium, especially as it relates to potassium, can cause problems. When sick with a flu or a cold, you lose sodium and should balance this by adding salt to what you eat. Sodium-enriched foods abound, including chicken broth, sports drinks, and canned beans and other vegetables. High amounts of sodium are usually listed on the ingredients labels of processed foods. Most women can obtain all the sodium their bodies need from whole foods without adding salt. If you frequently exercise heavily or perspire profusely, you may need to monitor your sodium intake to make sure you have enough. If you eat many canned foods, prepared dressings, processed foods, or packaged snack foods, or drink canned beverages, you may get an overload of sodium, however. High sodium can lead to high blood pressure, edema in pregnancy, arthritis, bloating, and some eye disorders. Sea salt is a natural salt and is recommended for the recipes in this book. ❧

setting goals

Now is the time to look back over your answers to the questions at the beginning of this chapter and set three goals for next week. Write three goals in your food diary. With each successive week you will be able to build on your goals and compare how you are today with how you were yesterday. Just observe and record how you feel and record your body's response to your healthy new snacking habits. It has taken you years to build up the unhealthy eating habits that deplete your energy. It won't take years to reverse those habits, but it will involve having realistic expectations about what you can change just for today or this week. For example, if you promise yourself you won't eat chocolate chip cookies for the entire week, even though you are used to eating them every day, you have set yourself up for failure. If, however, you tell yourself that your goal will be to eat five cookies instead of ten, or that your goal will be to eat dried fruits instead of the cookies one day each week, you will probably attain your goal.

chapter 7

healthy weight &
healthy hormones

Never give up, no matter what is going on, never give up. Too
much energy is spent developing the mind instead of the heart.
Be compassionate—not just to your friends, but to everyone, be compassionate.
Work for peace, and I say again, never give up, no matter what is happening, no
matter what is going on around you, never give up.
—Dalai Lama

we possess miraculously tuned bodies. Such a powerful
gift must be treated with great respect and even awe for the wisdom that
resides in every cell of our bodies. Maintaining a healthy weight should
be part of a lifelong commitment to celebrating your body.

healthy weight

How do you know if you have a healthy weight? Healthy weight depends
not on a weight chart but on you as an individual. It depends on your
lifestyle and culture, your bone structure, your personal happiness, and

whether or not you have symptoms of a hormonal imbalance that affects your metabolism. Do you want to keep your weight, or to lose or gain some pounds? Setting specific short-term and long-term goals is crucial to any endeavor, whether you're starting a busines or losing twenty pounds. To determine your weight goals, answer the following questions (if you want to maintain your current weight, skip them):

- *How much weight do you ultimately intend to lose or gain?*

- *How much weight do you want to lose or gain each week? (No more than one to two pounds, please.)*

- *How much weight do you want to lose or gain by the end of ten weeks?* ❧

use the food you eat

Our bodies have a natural instinct and ability to maintain balance. If given the chance, our bodies will naturally balance weight, energy, mood, and mental acumen. If we eat to balance our hormones, metabolism, weight, and digestion, we can live longer, age better, and feel that life is like a bowl of cherries. If we overload with fuel, our efficient bodies happily store it away in the form of fat to be used another day. Of course, most of us rarely need to use those stores, so we need to choose foods that do not add to our body's food storage and figure out ways to use stored food. The best way to rid the body of fat and excess weight is to exercise to burn the fuel and also to build muscle mass, which makes your body look thinner even if you don't lose much weight.

If you don't get enough activity, you need to find ways to increase it. Walk, ride a bicycle, visit your health club, go dancing. And exercise has another benefit for women hoping to balance their weight: the endorphins released during moderate to strenuous movement boost your mood and help prevent food cravings. Exercise helps release stress. Gentle exercise and deep breathing relieve fatigue. Stress and fatigue are primary factors in weight imbalance; they lead to depression and an inability to function, to think clearly, and to put our minds and bodies into action.

Stress, genes, environmental factors, lifestyle, and food choices actually can change our hormones. Hormonal fluctuation is what causes us to have symptoms including weight change. Whatever your weight concerns, the goal is to keep your hormones balanced.

This chapter will consider, primarily, the problems of hormonal imbalance affecting weight changes. But even if you are not concerned about weight, this is an important chapter for learning more about your body's needs. Eating that does not support the functioning of all of your glands may create a malfunction and can cause weight fluctuations at any time. ❧

weight gain during midlife

Many weight problems in midlife are related to natural hormonal changes that take place during and prior to menopause. Recent studies in the U.S. show some fat is essential for the storage of the vital hormones estrogen and progesterone. So, as the level of these hormones naturally decreases during and after menopause, it seems natural and healthy for women to gain some weight as they age as fat cells store the waning amounts of estrogen and progesterone. It is nature's way of keeping estrogen in the body for a longer time to keep women feeling young and to prevent aging symptoms.

Still, the possibility of gaining weight during menopause was the most serious concern of the five hundred American women who participated in my international survey at a women's health conference held at University of California Berkeley (Gaemi 1998). ❧

underweight or overweight: both are problems

Too much fat and too little fat are of equal significance to health, but the latter does not meet with the same alarm in a world where "you can never be too rich or too thin." There are anorexic girls in their teens who fill themselves up with water before being weighed by a doctor, women who have to be hospitalized because they diet themselves into near-fatal conditions, and dieting women who suffer hunger pangs, frustration, and depression, and spend thousands of dollars searching for the "perfect weight," which may not be their perfect weight at all. It is still the word "overweight" that strikes fear into the minds of the majority of women in America, even as the supersize fashion shops and fast-food promoters of the "double portion" thrive.

Some cultures do not value thinness, but value women with more flesh on their bones. In Egypt, very thin people are thought to be poor and incapable of feeding themselves. In traditional Hawaiian culture, people relished foods and enjoyed overeating—massaging their stomachs or having someone else massage their stomachs to aid digestion. These examples teach us to celebrate the joy of eating and the abundance of our world.

Of the influences that affect women's attitudes about weight, one of the most important is the media, which has helped to build a false image of women. All types of media are saturated with ads featuring young, underweight women, and it is difficult to escape the incessant suggestions that we must be slim to be attractive.

Specialty magazines and public television may offer good alternate information on healthy weight management but do not have the wide-reaching presence of publications and programs with massive commercial backing. This is an example of industry taking precedence over education. ❧

the role of the food industry

Women's obsession with staying thin has led to promotion of an endless variety of diet products. Some of these artificial and packaged convenience foods have actually manipulated our taste buds, so that we crave more fatty, salty, and sweet foods. Artificial sweeteners, for example, are 200 percent sweeter than natural sugar, and most research indicates that we can condition our body to prefer sweet foods. Some of us learn to love sweets from infancy. Long ago, our natural desire for sweets was helpful to enable us to gather fruits for nourishment, but now that so many of our sweets are made with refined sugar, our sweet tooth may not benefit our health.

Studies show that people who eat foods with artificial sweeteners tend to eat more to compensate for the lost calories. The Centers for Disease Control recently reported that U.S. obesity rates have gone up since NutraSweet was introduced and that 90 percent of dieters who lose weight regain all or part of it within five years, and of those who start commercial diet programs as many as 70 percent never complete them (Beck 2000).

Food labels are often misleading because consumers don't understand the implications or realize that chemical substitutes such as artificial sweeteners and partially hydrogenated oil are detrimental to our health. The problem with our lack of knowledge about food and health has kept us obsessed with weight without actually providing us with a method for sensible, healthy weight management. This is one of the reasons that Americans feel so depressed and guilty about weight. The stress of this depression and guilt is, ironically, yet another factor in the unhealthy diets of Americans, since stress can in turn lead to unhealthy eating.

Meanwhile, studies show Americans are getting fatter at an earlier age and about two-thirds of U.S. adults are overweight (Severson 2003). While Americans are buying more and more foods that contain artificial sweeteners and fat substitutes, they are gaining weight and complaining of low energy. The percentage of obese Americans is increasing rapidly. ❧

how you look at it

The media does not have the responsibility to solve diet problems, eating disorders, and individual weight problems. The responsibility for learning about healthy foods and eating habits, and incorporating them into a program for sensible weight management, is our own. The first step in changing our approach to nutrition is to become aware of how we have become captives to attitudes promoted by the media, the food industry, and our cultural eating habits.

The next step is explore and discover new practical processes that can transform these attitudes into ones that can improve not only our body's functioning but our moods as well.

JULIA'S STORY

Julia's one sincere enjoyment in life was that she had become a good gourmet cook. Julia was really almost obsessed with food and collected European dessert recipes. She impressed people by bringing elaborate desserts she made to parties, and having dinner parties with very elegant table settings.

She covered her size with clothes that were beautiful in texture and design, with interesting fabrics and expensive styling. She could accept her size the same way she accepted the lavish and decorative desserts she made that added to it. Her big problem with image was a skin problem that appeared as rashes on her face and body. Every time she looked in the mirror she felt diminished and depressed.

Julia had a family history of cancer and heart problems, hypo-glycemia, adult obesity, and diabetes and a personal history of obesity, weight fluctuations, yo-yo dieting, skin rashes with itching and burning, stress, thyroid problems, and chronic fatigue. She was not on HRT because of her other medical problems, and she did not want to be on it.

Julia was forty-eight years old when she became my client, and for the first time she admitted that food was her problem. She learned about hypoglycemia and that dependency on the wrong foods can be problem-atic, that eating habits are not inherited, and that healthy eating was in her power.

She began taking enzyme supplements, and she became interested in cooking and eating Asian and Middle Eastern foods. She had been using acupressure, but had never given thought to the culture from which it came. It was as if a whole new world opened up for her. She gained knowledge of yang and yin, low glycemic foods, high-chromium foods, the elements of food balance, and food variety, and through her discov-ery and exploration of spices, she became excited about food in a new way. Gradually, she changed from a fat-based to a spice-based way of cooking.

It was several months before she realized she no longer felt oppressed in her mind—no more mental fog or forgetting. Her skin cleared as her hypoglycemia got under control. She lost weight rapidly, then as her weight loss naturally became slower, she became more active and started getting massages and doing yoga and qigong.

Today, Julia is not the one to bring fancy desserts to gatherings, but she is praised and feels rewarded for her colorful, flavorful ethnic dishes and feels good because she knows she is doing something good for others, sharing healthy nutritious food that tastes wonderful.

Your goal is to choose foods based on your body-mind wisdom as discovered in your food diary, not based on trends. These are the foods that will satisfy your appetite while providing nutrients and balance. You are in control of your own food choices unless you relinquish that control, and by examining your reasons for the choices you make, you have the power to take charge. The food wisdom pyramid gives you a healthy alternative. ❧

taking control of your weight

Dieting is a common, and often unsuccessful, practice, as many women have learned from experience. It is a continuous cycle of losing and regaining weight. Losing muscle lowers the metabolism because muscle is metabolically active tissue.

Recent studies show that people who are overweight at forty have less life expectancy by at least three years than people who are underweight or are at a healthy weight. While a little excess weight can be protective because estrogen is stored in fat cells, obesity (over 25 percent of ideal body weight) can cause joint damage and make mobility a problem; put women at risk for diabetes and the resultant tissue damage; be a risk factor in heart disease and some cancers; and cause a higher risk of infection and poor wound healing, even when there is no indication that this is connected to an overall lowering of the immune function or overall poor health (American Institute for Cancer Research 2001).

Women who are underweight also suffer a number of problems. Most significantly, my underweight clients suffer more severe PMS, depression, and peri- and postmenopausal symptoms.

When you follow food wisdom, the person who needs weight will gain it and the person who needs to lose will lose because the body naturally adjusts to normal eating, not dieting. We have been taught to lose weight through dieting or to gain weight with supplements, but balanced eating is the healthiest way to achieve and maintain a healthy weight.

BODY IMAGE & YOUR HEALTHY WEIGHT

When we visualize ourselves as being at our healthiest, we imagine our skin being beautiful, our eyes bright, our energy high, our metabolism balanced, and our weight healthy. To reach this image of ourselves, we must turn to a wider variety of whole plant food: vegetables, seeds, and herbs.

The body's predilection for storing fat is an ancient biological phenomenon, and we need to educate ourselves about what is needed by the body for balance. When the body is satisfied and understands it will not go hungry or miss nutritional elements, it will balance its own weight. It will give you clues along the way as to how well you are feeding it. It will teach you to give yourself optimal care.

CULTURAL WISDOM OFFERS CLUES ABOUT LOSING WEIGHT

Although we can wait years for more research on what causes weight gain, we can start eating right and living balanced lives right away. Eating whole colorful plant foods for your body helps maintain a healthy weight.

Weight gain or loss is itself a symptom, and food wisdom looks at underlying causes and the mind-body of women rather than symptoms. For example, if your daily food diary shows you are exercising more yet still gaining weight, see if your eating patterns have changed. If your food intake has not changed, take a day for cleansing (see chapter 3). Women with concerns about their weight can often see a pattern in their food diary that may point to problems, such as diabetes, a lack of good digestive enzymes, hormonal imbalances, food sensitivities, or other underlying problems.

Cultural wisdom about losing weight, confirmed by modern research, suggests you should eat several small meals each day, avoid acidic or stressor foods (including excess high-fat, high-protein animal foods), eat breakfast, burn more calories than you consume by exercising, and cleanse your body with high-fiber and phytohormonal foods to make it better able to absorb nutrients. ❧

the glycemic index
& weight control

Controlling weight and health through hormonal balance depends on insulin resistance, dietary fiber, and the glycemic index of foods eaten. They are interrelated because they all have effects on sugar and insulin. Each food has a unique glycemic quality, which determines how quickly and for how long you will be energized by it. The glycemic content is affected by a food's fiber, protein, fat, and effect on blood sugar levels, and depends on the nutrient qualities of each food.

The Glycemic Research Institute's glycemic index (Ludwig 2002) shows foods that give more sustained energy, support better performance in athletes, limit sugar-related energy (high peaks followed by energy loss), and other hormonal imbalance symptoms, and can lower appetite and keep fat storage from accelerating. In addition, these foods help to prevent and control type 1 and type 2 diabetes and hypertension, hypoglycemia, and weight gain. This is because they are naturally low-fat, high-fiber foods. This research has been published in numerous nutrition journals and is supported by major health organizations such as the World Health Organization, the Canadian Diabetes Association, and the Food and Agriculture Organization.

The keys to glycemic balance are fiber, complex carbohydrates, protein, and essential fats, flavored with spices and herbs. When you eat high-sugar, high-starch, and low-fiber foods, it can cause insulin elevation and estrogen dominance or other hormonal imbalances, which are common in perimenopausal women and women with PMS. Fiber-rich foods and other low glycemic foods used daily can be invaluable for weight control, for a healthy thyroid, and for diabetes management. High-fiber foods take longer to chew, so you eat more slowly, and the chewing stimulates the production of saliva and other enzymes, which help you digest food more efficiently. High-fiber foods provide a way to eat large amounts of food while taking in relatively few calories. In addition, fiber absorbs water, making you feel fuller, so you eat less and feel satisfied longer. The body uses more calories to digest foods when you eat more complex carbohydrates and fiber.

Be sure to eat enough calories (not less than 1,200 per day) to prevent the body from reducing the metabolic rate at which calories burn. Remember, the body is constantly vigilant in its fierce determination not to let you starve to death. Follow the food wisdom pyramid. The following chart will give you an idea of the glycemic index for different foods (the index indicates how quickly and to what degree a carbohydrate-rich food raises blood sugar levels).

Glycemic Index (GI)	Food
High GI 100	glucose
80–99	baked potatoes, French bread, Corn Flakes, rice cakes, Rice Krispies, instant potatoes, pretzels
70–79	white rice, plain bagels, Cheerios, vanilla wafers, pumpkin, saltines, orange juice
Medium GI 60–69	whole grain bread, bran muffins, angel food cake, candy bars, pineapple, raisins, beets, rye bread
50–59	pasta, yams, bananas, oatmeal muffins, sweet potatoes, corn, popcorn, pears
Low GI 40–49	muesli, All-Bran cereal, bulgur, green grapes, peaches, apple juice, navy beans and baked beans, dried peas
30–39	garbanzo beans, pinto beans, black beans, dried prunes or plums, apples, low-fat milk, yogurt with fruit
20–29	lentils, pearl barley, kidney beans, grapefruit
10–19	plain yogurt, buttermilk, rice bran, soybeans

Tea can have a high glycemic index or low glycemic index, or neither, depending on what ingredients you add. Green tea, black tea, herbal teas and all my tea recipes in this book, for instance, tend to fall into the low glycemic index category.

Note: While diet sodas have no glycemic content, I strongly discourage drinking them until more studies are completed.

CHRISTINA'S STORY

Christina became severely fatigued and undernourished. Lack of fiber, phytohormonals, and essential fatty acids in a nonfat diet she was using was threatening her health. Essential fats are necessary to nourish and balance hormones and neurotransmitters. Christina was not losing weight, even though she was fanatically excluding fat from her diet. She ate a lot of simple carbohydrates, which were high glycemic foods, and so she was craving sweets. She was gaining weight from the calories in sugar.

She was also experiencing what many women consider to be common menopausal concerns: hot flashes, mood swings, and fatigue. Christina had never been told that these and other symptoms of hormonal changes might be a result of fluctuations in her blood sugar. Blood sugar that is either too high or too low is a problem, but too low means the body is in a state of hypoglycemia, which means you may feel shaky, have mood swings, and have food cravings and other health problems, as Christina did, which may lead to long-term weight concerns.

I explained to Christina that blood sugar changes hormone levels, such as insulin, and that frequent fiber snacking and eating small meals keep blood sugar stable and insulin balanced. Frequent snacking on medium and low glycemic index foods helped Christina find her individual balance level. She no longer allowed herself to reach the hunger stage, where her body became hypoglycemic. ❧

insulin resistance & chromium

For all people, but especially those with *insulin resistance* (when the body doesn't process insulin adequately), the key to maintaining a healthy weight and controlling insulin levels is to include enough chromium in the diet. Without adequate chromium intake, insulin does not work as well, bcause your cells are not as receptive to insulin's effect. The chromium-deficient individual has elevated blood sugar. Chromium is fundamental to blood sugar control and to prevent hypoglycemia.

Your chromium levels can get depleted if you eat too many refined sugars, because sugar increases chromium loss. White flour products may reduce your chromium intake because refined grains have chromium removed. Chromium deficiency has been linked to diabetes and coronary heart disease.

By now you should know that the best way to get enough chromium does not involve popping chromium pills. Instead, you can continue to focus on the food wisdom pyramid model, which provides a variety of medium to low glycemic index foods and high-fiber foods—fruits, greens, culinary herbs, olives, egg yolks, garbanzo beans, yogurt, alfalfa sprouts, beets, bitter melons, corn, apples, tomatoes, seaweed, kelp, and whole grains—all of which contain chromium. ✺

insulin & serotonin, the mood hormones

When you eat any carbohydrate (simple or complex), insulin is released. Ingestion of carbohydrates affects not only insulin, but also the brain hormone serotonin, which is responsible for mood control. Here's how it works: if you eat foods that are made of simple carbohydrates (high glycemic index), your blood sugar rises quickly and insulin is produced quickly. In addition, serotonin is produced immediately and the appetite is satisfied for a short period of time. Serotonin is directly responsible for the control of appetite and mood. We want serotonin to be produced gradually after a meal, so that our appetite can remain normal for an extended period of time. This occurs with a gradual increase in insulin levels that is consistent with a gradual increase in blood sugar, which only happens with high-fiber foods and other medium to low glycemic index foods.

Protein, fiber, and essential fats all slow a food's breakdown, while high glycemic foods, diet foods (such as artificial sweeteners), and some processed foods are broken down quickly. New research confirms that balancing one's levels of insulin and blood sugar can often control impulsive eating. Fiber has been proven to help control insulin release; therefore it is an important tool for weight and diabetes management.

In middle age, women face the added risk for adult-onset diabetes, uterine and breast cancer, and heart disease—all related to obesity. Recent studies show obesity and blood pressure are connected to levels of insulin. Insulin levels may be a major risk factor in heart disease in general because of the role it plays in the sympathetic nervous system. Insulin may increase risk for hypertension by increasing the rate of sodium retention in the body. Insulin tends to draw fat (lipids) from the blood stream and deposit it into fat cells. Therefore, too much insulin can lead to weight gain. 🪱

foods that help manage diabetes

Diabetes is a disease of the endocrine system connected to pancreas dysfunction. Type 1 diabetes, in which the pancreatic gland cannot produce adequate insulin, is genetic and is sometimes called juvenile diabetes. This type is present from an early age and those who have it are dependent on medically supervised insulin medication, used in conjunction with healthy eating and healthy weight, throughout their lives. Type 1 represents only a small percentage of the diabetes in this country.

Type 2, adult onset diabetes, is the more common type, and is related to diet, weight, attitude, and lifestyle. In America, type 2 diabetes is becoming an epidemic. Type 2 diabetes has increased as much as ten times over the past fifty years. Most people with type 2 diabetes have a high percentage of fat in their bodies (Lamendola 2003). In type 2, the body produces limited insulin, but high levels of glucose in the blood make it impossible for the insulin to do its job.

Both type 1 and type 2 diabetics can improve their health by eating medium to low glycemic foods and a diet high in fiber and low in animal fats, with a focus on herbs and spices such as licorice, fenugreek, and bitter melon. Using the cleansing way, maintaining a healthy weight and diet, and avoiding high glycemic and trigger foods will reduce your risk of becoming diabetic.

SYMPTOMS OF DIABETES

Symptoms can include any or all of these: sensations of tingling or numbness in hands or feet, blurry vision, frequent urination, extreme hunger, weight gain or loss, and recurrent skin, urinary tract, and vaginal infections. Diabetes is the leading cause of kidney disease. More than twice as many American women die from kidney disease as from breast cancer, but disfiguring breast cancer receives much more of the media's attention. Eating foods that help you feel full, speed up calorie burning, and block absorption and digestion of some dietary fat may reduce the risk of diabetes and facilitate its management (Lang et al. 1997).

Eat one medium fruit and a green salad at the beginning of every meal. This helps control blood sugar, and eating several small meals each day of high-fiber plant foods keeps insulin from fluctuating. Study the suggested dietary exchanges of the American Diabetic Association. The food wisdom pyramid offers freedom and creativity by substituting spices and herbs for sugar, salt, and fat. Carrying a travel snack is good planning. Exercise helps you to keep your metabolism moving and your weight balanced. In my practice, I have seen that foods high in chromium, including broccoli, beans, peanuts, and yogurt, may lower cravings for foods that cause weight gain, which increases diabetes risk.

DIABETES & SOLUBLE FIBER

A study conducted in West Africa, where no individual in a sampling of 1,381 had diabetes, helped nutritionists see that a low-fat diet high in fiber and complex carbohydrates could help diabetics (Teuscher et al. 1987). Soluble fiber, the type of fiber found in legumes such as soy, garbanzos, lentils, psyllium, fruits, vegetables, and oat bran and rice bran, forms a spongy mass in the intestines, releasing glucose slowly into the bloodstream. Studies have also shown that insufficient amounts of chromium, a trace mineral, may also be a factor. Eating foods high in chromium may decrease your chances of developing diabetes and help diabetics lower their craving for foods that cause weight gain or other stresses to their bodies (Mertz 1993; Bell and Goodrick 2002).

TESTING FOR DIABETES

Tests for diabetes are becoming a routine part of blood work, and you should be tested if you are over forty-five and are overweight or have a family history of diabetes (Karter 1996). Minorities are often more at risk, too, with diabetes afflicting 1.2 million Latino-Americans and 2.3 million African-Americans. Latino Americans are almost twice as likely to have the disease as non-Latino Caucasians, according to the Centers for Disease Control (Cimons 1997). Early detection can prevent complications such as heart disease, stroke, hypertension, hypothyroidism, and diseases of the eyes, kidneys, and nerves; these conditions result from the long-term effects of high glucose levels that characterize unbalanced eating's effect on diabetics. For more information on eating healthily with diabetes, see chapter 8.

WOMEN AT RISK

When some women consume high glycemic or refined-carbohydrate foods, they may experience one or more symptoms such as headaches, sweating, repeated need to urinate, cravings, mood swings, depression, or dehydration. These symptoms may indicate insulin resistance, a condition which may eventually lead to obesity and type 2 diabetes. Karen, a client who had a family history of type 2 diabetes, increased the amount of fiber she ate each morning when she was able to notice from her food diary that her headaches most often occurred after eating sweets. After a few weeks of following cleansing plan A (see chapter 3), the symptoms disappeared with no other treatment. By eating more foods with chromium, she was also able to lower her desire for sweets. She satisfied her sweet tooth with fruit.

Again, know what you are eating. Know what to avoid in packaged foods and how to read food labels, minimizing use of foods that list sugar in the first three ingredients, are high in fat, or have chemical additives. Concentrate on eating high-fiber foods, such as legumes, whole grain breads, fresh fruits, and vegetables. ❧

calcium & weight

Women who consumed 1,500 milligrams of calcium daily lost significantly more weight during a four year period, compared to a control group, according to a study from Creighton University's Osteoporosis Research Center (Zeml 2002). Calcium is important for metabolizing fat tissue to create energy and for storage of triglycerides. High-calcium foods, such as yogurt, buttermilk, kefir, feta cheese, tofu, tempeh, leafy greens, Jerusalem artichokes, culinary herbs, seaweed, sesame seeds, chicory, flaxseeds, and hummus, help to limit the accumulation of fat in your tissues and reduce the building of fat cells (Heaney, Davies, and Barger-Lux 2002). Better calcium absorption in the body has been linked to balanced insulin levels (Miller, Dunn, and Hachim 2003).

THE MIRACLE OF YOGURT

Yogurt, with its high protein, calcium, and magnesium content, may stabilize the immune system and metabolism, and lower blood cholesterol. Although more research is needed, microbiologists believe that yogurt with active cultures which helps the growth of good bacteria in the digestive system and may help eliminate toxins, even if the milk from which the yogurt is made was contaminated with hormones or pesticides (Ostman, Elmstahl, and Bjorck 2001). Women and men in Georgia and Gafghaz in Russia attribute a longer and more active life to eating yogurt (Gaemi 1975). A cup of low-fat cultured yogurt fortified with vitamin D contains 120 calories, 340 milligrams of calcium, and 11 grams of protein.

Buttermilk, a common beverage in the southern United States, is virtually watered-down yogurt, and contains all the live cultures and benefits of yogurt. To balance your acidity and alkalinity when using yogurt, you may add mint, honey, ginger, rose petals, raisins, or garlic.

So for healthy bones and healthy weight, focus on the bone food category of the food wisdom pyramid, follow the cleansing way chapter, eat high-fiber foods, and use high-quality-protein in recipes. ❧

tips for maintaining a healthy weight

- Limit high glycemic foods such as sugar, soda (including diet), highly concentrated sugar beverages, and refined bread, rice, and pasta (select whole grains and brown rice).

- Eat high-fiber whole foods, foods with calcium and chromium, and foods that aid calcium absorption (see chapter 1).

- Focus on aerobic exercises such as walking, bicycling, or swimming if your goal is burning fat.

- Choose at least some exercise where weights are lifted, such as lifting a heavy book in each hand, in order to build muscle.

- Improve flexibility and foster a sense of calm with yoga, qigong, and meditation.

- Meditate or write in your journal about self forgiveness.

- Eat a snack about a half hour before exercise. This will help your body burn more calories during the exercise than it would without the snack. Do not consume food or beverages other than water for one hour after exercise.

- No matter how hectic your morning schedule is, don't skip breakfast. Plan your breakfast the night before. In fact, make a habit of not skipping any meal, because your body may think you are starving, and your metabolism may slow down.

- Eat vegetables daily, especially greens, sprouts, and members of the cabbage family with root vegetables.

- For more protein, eat some egg whites, yogurt, almond butter, seaweed salad, and low-fat cheese such as feta, cottage cheese, ricotta cheese, and low-fat mozzarella cheese for breakfast or snacks.

- Eat one to two tablespoons daily of essential fatty acids from fish, flaxseeds, walnuts, or almonds.

LEILA'S STORY

Leila was in her late twenties and studying to be a psychologist when I met her. She was depressed and fat, smoked frequently, and found herself often bingeing on foods. Her self-image suffered, as she constantly asked herself who would come to her for therapy when they saw how unhealthy she looked. She was intelligent and people found her personality inviting, yet she had no confidence. "I hate cooking and nutrition. I don't even want to talk about it," she told me. She was eating mostly diet food, except for French bread. Her snacks were primarily diet soda, diet bars, and nonfat chips. She said her regimen made it easy for her: if it wasn't diet food, she didn't eat it. I gave her a list of snacking way choices and advised her to eat many diverse foods from the pyramid sections every day. I encouraged her to focus on medium to low glycemic index foods, and to take two lunch bags filled with phytohormonal foods with her to school and work each day. Hard-boiled eggs, pickled vegetables, cauliflower, fresh fruits, and sunflower seeds filled her bags. Eating these foods helped control her blood sugar and balance her neurotransmitters all day. When she arrived home at night, rather than being hungry and bingeing, she could calmly snack or eat a simple meal.

On my advice, Leila took an enzyme and multivitamin supplement with vitamins C and E, chromium, folic acid, iron, calcium, and magnesium. She adjusted to her new snacking way and said that eating no diet foods or starchy foods was easy now because her whole foods were now her favorite foods. She didn't miss the stressor foods. Eventually, using the food wisdom pyramid, Leila designed her own program. The foods Leila ate also balanced her moods and hormones, helping her feel good about herself. ❧

your thyroid gland's power over weight, life, & death

The life and death of our organs can depend on one small gland, the thyroid gland. This tiny gland at the base of your neck below your chin, nestled protectively in the groove of your collar bone, where you can rub or stimulate it and also guard it, is vital to the well-being of every part of your body. Often death is diagnosed as failure of the heart or some other organ, when, basically, it is the thyroid, seemingly silent and obscure, that has failed first, so that the other parts of the body dependent on it no longer have their life support.

Iodine, zinc, and copper are needed for effective thyroid hormone function. Iodine, zinc, and copper are found in plants that grow in nutrient-rich soil, and in many countries, including America, it is not necessary to use iodized salt. You can use sea salt, herbs, and spices for seasoning.

THYROID IMBALANCE

One of the first symptoms that may bring thyroid imbalance to your attention is weight gain. Estrogen tends to suppress thyroid gland function; imbalanced estrogen causes food to be stored as fat. Turning our stored body fat and the calories we eat into usable energy is a thyroid hormone function. Thyroid function also depends on the level of progesterone, which is, in turn, tied to estrogen levels.

In the cycle of interaction between thyroid and estrogen, low thyroid function and slow metabolism can mean an increase and imbalance of estrogen, and symptoms of *hypothyroidism*, also known as underactive thyroid, can often be mistaken for PMS, perimenopause, or menopause. Symptoms of hypothyroidism include fatigue, depression, insomnia, puffy face, constipation, cold or numb hands or feet, chills, painful or excessive menstrual periods, memory loss, excess of white hair, dry or scaly skin, and lower sex drive. Another symptom of low thyroid function is low body temperature, which occurs because the sympathetic nervous system may be affected when peripheral blood vessels are not getting a balance of nutrients to the thyroid gland. And if peripheral blood vessels constrict in response to stress or fear, blood flow to the body's surface is reduced.

Hyperthyroid means the gland produces too much thyroid hormone. Weight loss, weakness, high blood pressure, and a shaky feeling or actual trembling of the hands are symptoms, as are, in extreme cases, bulging eyes and the development of a goiter.

Potential causes of thyroid imbalance are autoimmune inflammation and stress. To help manage your stress, use breathing meditations, movement, qigong, and exercise, which can increase circulation to the thyroid.

Support the thyroid gland by eating hormonally. Eat antioxidant foods and whole grains, and avoid trans fats and fatty meats. Note in your food diary your response to cabbage, broccoli, radishes, or cauliflower; these can induce goiter formation and can interfere with thyroid function, but in general are needed to support your hormones.

The Thyroid Foundation of America (www.tsh.org) gives free, up-to-date information on preserving glands and metabolic balance through hormone secretion, and the latest approaches to treating goiter, thyroiditis, hyperthyroidism, hypothyroidism, and nodules, tumors, and cancers involving the thyroid gland as well as lymphoma, involving the lymph glands. If you think you have a thyroid imbalance, see your physician. ✌

food wisdom prescription for a healthy weight

Look to food wisdom if you are troubled by weight gain. You can also use the following plans.

The cleansing way: Use cleansing plan A (see chapter 3) for two or three days each week to achieve and maintain a healthy weight. If you experience excess cravings, weight gain, indigestion, or fatigue, switch to plan B for food sensitivities.

Snacking and morning way: See chapters 4 and 6 for ideas on breakfast and snacking. Chew on fresh tarragon, mint, basil, cilantro, cucumber, lettuce, bitter melon, endive, and dill all day. Sip on miso and yogurt soup. Carry healthy snacks with you everywhere.

Tea way: Drink green tea (morning), black tea (afternoon), fruit and flower tea (Healthy and Wise Tea). Add sweet spices such as licorice, cinnamon, cayenne, and cloves in winter and anise and mint in summer. Treat yourself to a chai soy latte, cold or warm. Snack on ginger and natural licorice candy, raisins, and fresh fruits.

Movement way: Use daily breathing, visualizations, and relaxation exercises. Practice breathing well any time of day for any length of time. Exercise three times a week or as your schedule allows three to five hours per week. A support group for movement helps many, but the bottom line is that your own body will be giving you responses to your choices: write your movement statement and goals in your food diary: list activities you enjoy, when and why you move, what you eat, and how food and exercise make you feel.

Lifestyle way: Eat at least five to six small meals including snacks each day. For one week eat watermelon, salad, greens, and culinary herbs before every meal. Eat an early, low-protein dinner. Planning has priority in maintaining weight and weight loss; plan for shopping, bag lunches, portable snacks, and eating out, so you can make wise food choices. Be aware to be thankful for food flavors, for colors, for the qualities of healthfulness in food. Understand your food sensitivities and think of the cultural patterns that influence you and shape your life. Be proud to accept yourself, your weight and appearance. Create surroundings for your relaxation, comfort, inspiration, and aesthetic pleasure. Create affirmations for yourself through self-improvement tapes, videos, and books.

chapter 8

preventing & relieving major symptoms of hormonal imbalances

West is focusing on replacing and East is focusing on restoring, and food therapy will bridge East and West, just as it is the paradigm that is bridging science and tradition.
—Sonia Gaemi, Ed.D., RD

if you are eating hormonally, your symptoms from hormonal imbalance will disappear over time, and your body will grow stronger. Food wisdom healing therapy also offers specific prescriptions, therapeutic eating plans including teas, snacking, and breakfast ideas, lifestyle ideas, movement, breathing, and other advice for specific body-mind conditions. The more food therapy practices you follow regularly, the better your health will be. ❧

food wisdom prescriptions

The following prescriptions for different conditions are based on food pyramid balance and food wisdom ways. The prescriptions relate to and depend on all of the healing ways in this book. Always consult your health care provider before beginning any new food regimen.

ALLERGIES OR FOOD SENSITIVITIES

At least 50 percent of Americans suffer from food sensitivities, or allergies, which can affect you emotionally, mentally, and physically and vary from person to person, causing asthma, depression, skin rashes, eczema, hives, indigestion, excess mucus, colitis, insomnia, weight gain, headaches or migraines, or other symptoms. Allergic reactions come from the immune system acting on a specific protein, immunoglobulin E (IgE), in the blood, causing the body to release a flood of chemicals such as histamine, which cause allergic symptoms. See your physician for allergy testing or try cleansing plan B.

Food Therapy for Allergies or Food Sensitivities

Marta, with severe fatigue, headaches, and insomnia, used cleansing plan B and the elimination process, which helped her discover that she could no longer use soy. She checked the food pyramid and chose other legumes to have instead, such as garbanzo and black beans, which gave her the nutritional value of soy without causing problems for her. At the time, she did not know the scientific basis for her food sensitivity, but soon learned that too much isolated soy protein may inhibit the transfer of glucose to the brain. Later I told her to introduce very small amounts of a fermented form of soy, such as fermented tofu, miso, or tempeh, into her system on occasion, because when foods are partially digested by bacteria in the fermentation process, they become easier to digest. She was then able to get the benefits of soy without symptoms.

> **Food therapy way:** Start your food therapy with cleansing plan A to accustom your body to the omission of high stressor foods, and after two to three weeks switch to plan B to trace common or specific foods to which you may be sensitive.

Colors: Black and white to support lungs, kidneys, and colon, which are the most important organs in terms of food allergies.

Specific prescription: Five to seven mornings a week, take 2 tablespoons each of Sophia's Seeds (see chapter 3 for formula) and/or ground flaxseeds and 1 teaspoon each of anise seeds and honey, add 1 cup or more of hot water, and drink. Or drink a glass of blended mixed beets and cilantro (one medium beet and 2 cups of cilantro), adding a pinch of anise and cayenne pepper in the blender.

Foods to increase: Foods high in magnesium (amaranth, brown rice), iron (green leafy foods, organic liver, raisins), B vitamins (beans and legumes), bioflavonoids (onions, garlic, citrus fruits including the white membrane), cilantro, turmeric, olives, parsley, buckwheat, black currants, and red and black grapes.

Morning and snacking way: Sophia's Energizing Lentil Cereal (see chapter 4) with lime, buckwheat, amaranth, and soy or almond milk; white- or black-color Sonia's Antioxidant Smoothie (see chapter 10); yogurt mixed with tropical fruits such as kiwi, passion fruit, and papaya (except pineapple which is acidic or very yang in Chinese medicine).

Tea way: Any tea in chapter 5 or black currant tea.

Lifestyle: Conscious breathing. Write in your food diary.

Supplements: Extra enzymes, vitamin C, and multivitamins.

Complementary and folk favorites: Aloe vera juice, licorice, or slippery elm in your tea.

ANEMIA & FATIGUE

Many women experience fatigue related to anemia. This can be related to lack of iron, healthy enzymes, vitamin B_{12}, folic acid, and vitamin E. Iron forms hemoglobin, which carries oxygen, and thus when blood is lost monthly, more hemoglobin, must be manufactured, requiring more iron. Without enough iron, oxygen does not reach the brain and cells, and you grow tired.

Food therapy way: Use cleansing plan A one to three days weekly. Eat medium to low glycemic foods.

Colors: Green, red.

Foods to increase: Pistachios, assorted leafy green lettuce, and organic liver (2 ounces two or three times monthly). Try making omelets and soups using greens, such as turnip greens, spinach, dandelion greens, purslane, poke greens, or mustard greens, or try arugula with yogurt with added brewers yeast (1 teaspoon per meal). Moreover, try to increase your intake of foods that are high in vitamin C when eating iron-rich foods, such as meat, for it will increase your absorption of iron.

Morning and snacking way: Start each morning with water and a papaya or pear. Add pistachios and prunes to your iron-fortified cereal. Also recommended are citrus fruits, cantaloupe, dried fruits, toasted seaweed, and tomatoes.

Tea way: If you are eating iron-rich meals, don't drink black tea or coffee with the meal, as the polyphenols found in these drinks will inhibit iron absorption by as much as 70 percent. Herbal tea with lime, berries, and culinary herbs increases absorption of iron.

Lifestyle: Meditation and exercise will increase oxygen and help to balance yin and yang. Get frequent and good sleep and rest. Cook foods in copper and iron pots.

Supplements: Your daily supplement may include liquid iron, extra enzymes, folic acid, vitamin C with rose hips, and Siberian ginseng.

Complementary and folk favorites: Use blackstrap molasses in cereal, yogurt, and dressings, and in baking.

ARTHRITIS OR OSTEOARTHRITIS

Arthritis is a degenerative joint disease characterized by inflammation at a point where bones join together. Double-blind studies show that between 85 and 90 percent of patients with symptoms of arthritis react to certain foods. Several lifestyle and food sensitivities may adversely affect arthritis. Too much iron and circulating calcium that does not become bone may be a factor. Hormonal imbalance, especially in women with PMS or menopause symptoms, environmental factors, strain from physical activity, which can create joint and muscle pain, and excess weight that puts stress on your bones can all contribute.

Food therapy way: Use cleansing plan A twice a week for a month, then switch to plan B and check for food sensitivity. Steam your food. Eat medium to low glycemic foods.

Colors: Green, brown, yellow, red.

Specific prescription: Eat 3 to 5 cloves of garlic a day or Aged Garlic (see chapter 10); take 2 teaspoons each ground flaxseed and organic turmeric daily, sprinkled on your foods. Try fish baked with walnut, garlic, ginger, turmeric, and other yang spices.

Foods to increase: Studies show that omega-3 fatty acids, found in cold-water fish, such as herring, sardines, salmon, and mackerel, reduce inflammation and pain. Walnuts mixed with cilantro may have a similar effect. Increase yang spices. Substitute plant protein instead of animal protein: garbanzos, soybeans, red beans, mung beans, purslane, barley, buckwheat, pecans, walnuts, and flaxseeds.

Avoid all triggers: Especially wheat, dairy (milk and cheese) and other animal foods, and members of the nightshade plant family, such as tomatoes, eggplant, peppers, and potatoes. Pay attention to environmental triggers such as dampness, humidity, and smoking.

Morning and snacking way: Make Sonia's Antioxidant Smoothies (see chapter 10), adding 1 cup cilantro, 1 tablespoon each of chopped figs, pistachios, crystallized ginger, raisins, dried fruit, seeds, and nuts, and a pinch of cardamom seeds and cinnamon.

Tea way: Chai latte with soy milk; tea with ginger, cinnamon, angelica, or licorice added.

Lifestyle: Sun therapy and breathing therapy; acupressure; controlled movement such as walking, qigong, tai chi, or yoga; swimming; if possible visit, dry, hot climates and use dry saunas. If you swim or participate in water exercise often, you might want to eat extra ginger, garlic, and turmeric to counteract the humidity. Massage ginger, sesame oil, or eucalyptus oil into joints. A cayenne or turmeric wrap (a warm cloth saturated with turmeric and flaxseed oil) may ease pain or discomfort by stimulating blood flow to the area.

Supplements: Multivitamin (200 percent DV), vitamin E (800 IU), vitamin C (2000 mg), 2 to 3 turmeric capsules, and 2 to 3 enzyme supplements.

Complementary and folk favorites: Acupuncture, pressure point massage, or reflexology for energy circulation. Add corn silk, parsnip, black cohosh, kava kava, or cayenne pepper to teas. There are reports that white willow bark works as well as aspirin. Use of glucosamine (as a supplement) may protect cartilage and relieve arthritis; consult with your doctor.

Note: These suggestions are based on a sense of coldness in your joints. If you feel heat or pain in your joints or muscles, or see redness and swelling, you may need to balance with cooling yin foods and cooling climate.

CONSTIPATION & IRREGULARITY

Cleansing plan A is a foundation for having healthy bowel movements. Start your morning with a pear or 3 to 5 prunes and fiber such as Sophia's Seeds (see formula in chapter 3) with an extra 2 to 3 cups of water. Throughout the day use high-fiber snacking. Add 1 tablespoon grape seed oil or olive oil or flaxseeds to leafy greens. Apply aloe vera gel to relieve the discomfort or itching of hemorrhoids, or sit in a tub of warm water.

Fatigue is a complex problem, but in many cases it may be caused by constipation. Cleansing plans A and B, based on high fiber and complex carbohydrates, cleanse your system naturally for more energy.

DIABETES

The food therapy way for diabetes management is designed to help diabetics manage their blood sugar through the food they eat, as well as through positive lifestyle changes. According to the Centers for Disease Control, one in three children born in 2000 will develop type 2 diabetes due to unhealthy eating habits and increasing obesity unless Americans change their lifestyles to include healthier foods and more physical activity (McConnaughey, 2003).

Food therapy way: Use cleansing plan A once or twice a week.

Colors: Use different colors of vegetables and fruits each day: yellow for Monday, white for Tuesday, and so on.

Specific prescription: Eat five or six small meals each day; be sure to eat 1 medium piece of fruit with every meal.

Foods to increase: Fiber, fruit, fenugreek, licorice, bitter melon, cabbage, alfalfa, turnip, coriander seeds, garlic, barley bread, and foods high in chromium.

Morning way: Oatmeal, Sonia's Phytoestrogenic Cereal (see chapter 4) with rice bran and fenugreek powder (1 teaspoon).

Tea way: Healthy & Wise Tea or Denna's Herbal Chai. See my other recipes in chapter 5.

Lifestyle: Visit the American Diabetic Association Web site (www. diabetes.org) for ideas about positive lifestyle changes you can make to help manage diabetes.

Supplements: Multivitamins and extra enzymes; for menopausal and postmenopausal women, choose a multivitamin without iron. Take bilberry to protect your eyes.

DEPRESSION & ANXIETY

With as many as 12 million people in the United States suffering from depression and the number seemingly rising, we need to be aware of the symptoms. The complexity of our brains and our emotional lives makes problems such as depression difficult to heal.

Depressed people usually have lower levels of neurotransmitters such as serotonin. All serotonin used by the brain must be manufactured in the neurons, and the production of serotonin is dependent on the presence of amino acids LT and tryptophan, which seem to transport the serotonin into the brain. Stress can lower the presence of both these compounds in the body. Another type of depression is seasonal affective disorder, or SAD. In darker seasons, people with SAD find themselves fatigued, craving sweets or starches, and sleeping more. Lack of sunlight causes too much production of melatonin, and may decrease levels of the neurotransmitter serotonin, which influences moods.

Deficiency of folic acid can lead to depression. Stress, hormonal fluctuations, and oral contraceptives may leach folic acid from the body.

Causes of depression can also include environmental and/or nutritional factors. Certain foods, intense color, certain smells, antioxidants, and phytonutrients can balance moods and create a feeling of well-being. Your doctor, therapist, or other health professional may be able to work with a dietitian or a food therapist to determine whether your depression is caused by an underlying health condition or situational factors.

If you have symptoms such as loss of energy, inactivity, fatigue, feelings of sadness, emptiness, guilt and helplessness, irritability, anxiety, loss of sense of smell or taste and appetite, weight issues or eating disorders, you may be suffering from depression. Alcohol, smoking, caffeine, sleeping pills, and high glycemic foods (such as sugary, starchy foods) and low fiber foods may contribute to depression. Balancing hormonal fluctuations by balancing neurotransmitters in the brain can steady moods. Creating a healthy body can be the start of healing depression and other mood disorders. Taking a weekly cleansing day, eating from the food wisdom pyramid, and taking time out for breathing, movement and meditation can help ease the symptoms of depression. Visit your mental health professional before beginning any new treatment for depression, and get help immediately immediately if you feel suicidal.

DIARRHEA

Use foods easy on your digestive tract. Foods with pectin can be helpful: applesauce or steamed apple (no skin), rice, barley, steamed sweet potatoes, and carrots. Use bananas, apricots, and mashed potatoes to replenish potassium. Use fat-free chicken broth or miso and seaweed to replenish protein and sodium. For severe diarrhea, ginger ale helps balance lost sugar.

GASTROINTESTINAL PROBLEMS

Poor digestion can undermine the immune system, and a healthy immune system, healthy good bacteria, and healthy hormones will determine the health of your gastrointestinal system. Good digestive bacteria are the foundation of a healthy digestive system. When digestion and absorption are healthy, generally you will not have gastrointestinal complications, such as colitis, diverticulitis, irritable bowel syndrome, or leaky gut syndrome, and symptoms such as bad breath, gas, or bloating.

A tip: Something as simple as drinking liquids during meals may dilute your digestive enzymes, so for better digestion use liquids after or before meals.

Tibetan medicine tradition encourages watermelon (or dried fruits such as berries, apricots, peaches, or pears soaked with juice when watermelon is not in season) before a meal or as a appetizer. This cleans up the heat (too much yang food residue) from the digestive tract.

Food therapy way: Use cleansing plan A for three to four days per week. Focus on medium to low glycemic foods.

Colors: Yellow, golden, green, and white.

Specific prescription: Eat five to six small meals daily; increase fiber daily with seeds and/or 1 to 2 tablespoons of psyllium husk (unless your doctor wants you take a powder form); and increase herbs (½ cup fresh tarragon, mint, rosemary, or thyme) in a salad or yogurt. Three times per week, steam 1 cup of parsley with 1 cup of water for twenty minutes and drink the juice before a meal or mix the cooked parsley with tofu or yogurt. Enjoy fruits and vegetables such as kiwi, papaya, Asian pear, baked squash, or yams an hour before a meal for enzyme stimulation. Most cultures use fruit as an appetizer or snack before meals to stimulate healthy digestion. To prevent indigestion, bloating, or gas, sprinkle marjoram, anise, or fennel on your beans or vegetables. Your food therapy journal will help you understand what combination of fruit and protein works best for your own good digestion.

Foods to increase: Brown rice syrup, barley malt syrup, or raw honey in your smoothies can aid digestion or lessen allergy symptoms. Add yogurt and culinary herbs such as mint. Add 1 tablespoon of 5 percent apple cider vinegar to your soup or salad at noon.

Avoid all triggers: Stress, stressor foods, missing meals.

Tea way: Tea soothes and calms the digestive system. Drink tea 20 minutes before and after each meal. Add thyme, mint, ginger, fennel, fenugreek, licorice, and cloves to your tea.

Morning and snacking way: Buckwheat and kashi cereal with yogurt, Sonia's Antioxidant Smoothie (see chapter 10), snacks high in protein, juice from fermented wheat, or wheat berry sprouts.

Lifestyle: Check your environment, your food, and your stress. Consult your doctor for your progesterone and estrogen ratio level. Most women complain of gastrointestinal problems when they experience hormonal imbalance. Smoking and alcohol contribute to malabsorption. Chew raw and whole foods to stimulate digestive enzymes.

Supplements: Take extra enzymes and multivitamins with meals to increase absorption. Capsules of turmeric mixed with ginger, one per meal, soothe inflammation and irritabilities.

Complementary and folk favorites: Marshmallow (the herb, not the candy), black cohosh, slippery elm bark, or horsetail grass tea. Licorice root tincture (chopped or powder) in tea is the herb Middle Eastern women are using (if you have high blood pressure, consult with your doctor or health professional).

PREMENSTRUAL SYNDROME (PMS)

If you suffer from PMS, use your food diary, recording and rating any symptoms, both physical and emotional, that you have throughout the month. Be sure to record foods, mood swings, cravings, and symptoms. Rate them from 1 (the best) to 10 (the worst).

Food therapy way: Use cleansing plan A one day each week (or more, as needed). Focus on medium to low glycemic foods.

Colors: Red, green, and brown.

Specific prescription: Drink daily Sonia's Antioxidant Smoothie (see chapter 10) with red and green foods and added rice bran and roasted garbanzo flour (1 to 2 tablespoons) and flaxseeds (2 to 3 tablespoons). For a week before your period, rest more and eat simple foods (limit fried, creamy, and spicy foods, and foods which you have found give you gas). Eat five to six small meals daily to ease your digestive and hormonal system.

Foods to increase: Foods high in magnesium (garbanzos, parsley, cilantro, broccoli, amaranth, buckwheat, almonds, roasted seaweed), potassium (kiwis, beets), vitamin B_6 (bananas, potatoes with skin, winter squash, seafood, prunes, oatmeal), boron (berries, prunes, peaches, grapes, tomatoes, apples, pears), and vitamin E (almonds, sunflower seeds).

Morning and snacking way: Roasted buckwheat, yogurt, Tonic Pears (see chapter 10), baked potatoes, millet toast with tofu cheese and sliced papaya, fresh cilantro or mint, fresh or dried fruit, berries, sunflower seeds, bananas, almonds, pumpkin seeds, beans, baked yams, freshly squeezed juice with cilantro, raw cauliflower or broccoli, baby cucumber.

Tea way: During your period, drink tea with a minimum of tea leaves to avoid caffeine. Add mint, berries, borage, rose petals, dandelion, clover, cranberry, pomegranate, blueberries, barberry, angelica, and hibiscus.

Recipe way: Sasha's Mood Burritos, Noble High-Energy Garbanzo Pilaf, Calming Persian Cold Yogurt Soup (see chapter 10); hummus; steamed red endive sprinkled with cinnamon; bean soups and stews.

Lifestyle: Keep your body warm during and before your periods. Tea becomes part of this lifestyle, especially Denna's Herbal Chai. Rest before and during your period. A warm bath with lemongrass (tied in cheesecloth) may calm PMS symptoms. Use this acupressure point to relieve menstrual cramps: Press your thumb on the inside of your ankle between the anklebone and the heel. Then press your index finger on the same area on the outside of your ankle. Women taking oral contraceptives should eat foods high in B vitamins, such as cabbage, grains, yogurt, split peas, nuts, legumes, and fennel seeds, to alleviate mood swings or fatigue.

Supplements: Extra enzymes, multivitamins (150 percent of DV), vitamin C (1000 milligrams), vitamin B_6 (4 milligrams; 200 percent

DV), kelp capsules. Wheat germ or its oil is high in essential fats and also is high in vitamin E.

Complementary and folk favorites: Barberry, dong quai (angelica), and bearberry—but only for short time. According to some herbalists, dong quai has a balancing effect on estrogen. Drink motherwort tea two to three times daily when you feel cramps. Black cohosh has become popular with menstruating and menopausal women because of its phytohormonal properties. American Indians used it to treat women's menstrual problems and rheumatism. (Pregnant women should not use black cohosh, however, as it can stimulate menstrual flow and cause severe complications.)

HEADACHES & MIGRAINES

Migraines as well as headaches and cramping may be totally nutritionally related symptoms and most women can use food choices to prevent them. If you have severe migraines, see your doctor. Using your food diary and cleansing plan B is the best way to learn if food sensitivities, yeast, common allergenic foods, or other stressors are the cause of the symptoms. A deficiency of iron, vitamin E, folic acid, or other nutrients may be a cause. Eating small snacks several times a day prevents hunger and keeps your blood sugar balanced. Take extra vitamin C (2000 milligrams) with rose hips, or drink rose hip tea as it contains bioflavonoids combined naturally with vitamin C. Take enzyme supplements, multivitamins, and folic acid. Inhale the scent of rosemary, use it in cooking and tea, and massage the oil onto your ears and neck. Reflexology is often beneficial. Use the suggestions in the cleansing chapter. Angelica or feverfew as a tea may help relieve a headache.

PREVENTING CANCER & SUPPORTING RECOVERY

Science has completed many studies regarding specific foods and their relevancy to specific cancers. Primary in boosting your immune system are protein, antioxidants, enzymes, and fiber, which stimulate the immune system to produce antibodies to protect cells from cancer (Rao 2000). By eating delicious plant proteins such as tofu, black beans, and hummus, you can avoid the high levels of fat from animal protein. There is some question about the phytoestrogen content of soy and its effect on cancer patients, but sufficient research has not been done on this topic. However, the cultural practice of using fermented soy as Asians do has been proven healthy for centuries. My advice is to eat soy in its fermented forms, such as tofu, tempeh, and miso, and eat it in moderation.

Food therapy way: Follow the food wisdom pyramid and cleansing plan A. Focus on medium to low glycemic foods.

Colors: Yellow, pink, red, purple.

Specific prescription: Seeds every morning and 1 to 2 cups of antioxidant fruits such as oranges, berries, grapes, or dried or fresh prunes before meals. Eat daily 1 to 2 cups of dark green salad such as parsley, arugula, spinach, watercress, cruciferous vegetables (cabbage, mustard, turnips, broccoli, kale). Three to four times weekly blend ginger, garlic, yogurt, and mint, or eat hummus, mushrooms, or corn.

Morning and snacking way: Melon and papaya slices in corn or rice cereal; Sonia's Antioxidant Smoothies (see chapter 10) with blueberries, prunes, 1 to 2 egg whites, and flaxseeds; carrot juice with ginger; dried cranberries and sesame seeds; popcorn; Roasted Garbanzo Beans; and Boshki's Travel Snack (see chapter 6).

Tea way: Green or mint tea with ginseng, licorice, borage, and hibiscus.

Lifestyle: Cleansing for detoxification of environmental toxins is very powerful, as is conscious deep breathing. Qigong, yoga, and movement will help you with a healthy weight balance and keep your mood elevated while you follow food therapy. Get plenty of rest and sleep, and use meditation and visualizations to affirm your choice of positive health. In chemotherapy or recovery, an important thing in healing is appetite; even if all you yearn for is cheese salami pizza, eat and enjoy some! A food and feelings diary is also a vital tool.

Supplements: Organic enzyme supplements and a multivitamin with antioxidants, vitamin C, and IP6 antioxidant supplement taken with meals.

Complementary and folk favorites: Aloe vera juice in a shake, or echinacea root, goldenseal, Siberian ginseng, American ginseng, and elderberry as tea.

HAIR LOSS

Hair loss can be triggered by allergies, food sensitivities, stress, emotional factors, nutritional deficiencies, reaction to medication or supplements used inappropriately, or environmental toxins. Hair loss can be caused by an imbalance of progesterone. Check with your physician to rule out this possibility. Increase fiber foods and use cleansing plan A to cleanse the system. Drink 1 to 3 teaspoons of blackstrap molasses in a cup of warm water one to three times a day. A folk method to increase hair growth is to rub hazelnut or almond oil on your scalp, leave it on overnight, and shampoo. Many conditioners now contain mango and other antioxidant foods; leave conditioner on clean hair.

HEART PROBLEMS

Heart disease is the number one cause of death among women. Risk factors for heart disease include diabetes, previous heart attack, angina, heart failure, lack of exercise, uncontrolled high blood pressure, high cholesterol, and kidney problems.

Food therapy way: For preventing heart problems or for healing or reversing heart disease, combine foods from the food wisdom pyramid with cleansing plan A. Focus on medium to low glycemic foods.

Colors: Intense red, purple, gold, and green.

Specific prescription: Eat daily 1 cup roasted or cooked garbanzo beans, lentils, or tofu (interchangeably) and 1 cup berries and red or black grapes (can be used in daily tea); ½ cup fresh dill with lunch or in smoothies (add 2 tablespoons each soy bran, roasted garbanzo flour, and flaxseeds), and cold water. Eat fish two to three times per week. Use strongly flavored oil for cooking. Read food labels for stressor foods (omit trans-fatty acids or hydrogenated oils); check ingredients of processed foods. Substitute yin and yang spices for salt, fat, and sugar.

Foods to increase: Calming Persian Cold Yogurt Soup (see chapter 10), Sonia's Energizing Lentil Cereal (see chapter 4), pomegranate or grape juice. Eat an early, light dinner, such as bread with hummus and basil, or with grapes, walnuts, almonds, feta cheese, and olives.

Tea way: 2 cups of black tea (if you are menopausal) with ginger or dill; Wise Flower Tea (chapter 5).

Lifestyle: For managing stress: spend time in nature or viewing nature. Plant trees and garden. Studies show that having a pet comforts and relaxes the body, while loneliness increases heart problems. Do cardiovascular exercise (any nonstrenuous exercise that increases your heartbeat). A small amount of red wine—not more than half a glass per night—has been shown to be beneficial for the heart. When you eat high-fiber plant foods, you can safely eat 1 to 3 eggs per week if desired.

Supplements: Multivitamin with antioxidants, folic acid (400 to 700 milligrams), Q-10 enzyme, organic chlorophyll, and enzymes.

Complementary or folk favorites: Hawthorn, black cohosh, and vitex tincture, which stimulates natural estrogen production. In the Middle East, valerian, borage, and dried lemon (1 teaspoon each) are widely used as a tea.

HIGH BLOOD PRESSURE

When you eat for your heart, bones, and hormones, the nutrients take care of high blood pressure, so follow the plan for a healthy heart. Eating whole plant foods, including a variety of seeds, nuts, grains, fruits, and vegetables and cutting down on stressor foods, especially high glycemic index foods, animal fat, and trans-fatty acids, is the key to lowering high blood pressure. The bone foods that help lower blood pressure include potassium foods, such as beet greens, avocado, apricots, and beets. These contain high amounts of potassium and may even lower the amount of medication women with high blood pressure need. Calcium- and magnesium-rich foods help the body relax and eliminate excess sodium, and may help lower blood pressure. The natural salt in many whole plant foods can supply the salt your body needs. Sumac powder (found in Middle Eastern stores) is a delicious red spice traditionally used as a salt substitute. Be aware that research shows licorice increases high blood pressure. Focus on Cleansing Plan A and on medium to low glycemic foods. A menu that emphasizes high fiber and is high in essential fats and low-fat dairy products may act as a natural diuretic that could help many people reduce blood pressure without the use of medication, according to a recent report (Michalkiewicz et al. 2003).

COMPLICATIONS FROM HYSTERECTOMY

Women sometimes have hysterectomies to correct uterine bleeding, pelvic pain, endometriosis, fibroids, or a prolapsed uterus, though medical management of these conditions may be preferable. Women who have sexual problems or a higher rate of depression or anxiety before a hysterectomy may have the same problems afterward.

Hysterectomies are not the only option. Eating hormonally, with precise supplementation, can activate your body to begin to heal itself. The healing process can be hastened by stimulation of acupressure points and also by engaging in spiritual practice.

INSOMNIA

For seven consecutive days, list major and minor stresses in your food diary. Include the foods you've eaten and how you felt after eating them. Learn to clarify your feelings to yourself; you will then be able to seek a solution. Have your doctor watch your estrogen and progesterone ratio if you have insomnia or anxiety.

Food therapy way: Focus on high-selenium foods and cooling yin spices. Eat foods containing tryptophan to help you relax. These include hummus; a turkey sandwich with seeds and greens; low-fat yogurt mixed with cucumber, seaweed, pumpkin seeds, and sunflower seeds; soy and nut milks; and kelp. Although sugary foods and alcohol such as wine may initially make you feel drowsy, these foods can cause wakefulness later in the night. It's best to limit them in the evening.

Tea way: Herbal tea without caffeine, used all day and evening, relieves stress. Add passionflower, peppermint, borage, chamomile, hops, and kelp to your desired tea or tea bag.

Lifestyle: Limit smoking or consuming caffeine and sugary beverages after lunch. Eat an early dinner of plant foods, light on protein.

- Meditate or do visualization exercises before retiring. Listen to soothing music.

- Walk for 10 to 15 minutes after dinner—often some fresh air and a short walk in a protected area will help women find restful sleep.

- Counting when you wake up in middle of night puts you back to sleep.

- Rub the insomnia acupressure points in your feet (2 inches in from you heel).

- Go to a sauna, jacuzzi, or hot tub in the evening, or take a warm or shower or bath and spray orange blossom water all over yourself for aromatherapy before going to bed.

- If you feel bombarded by information all day and find yourself running through bits of this mental noise as you try to fall asleep, write down your thoughts that are most important, and let the rest disappear. You do not need to know or do everything.

- Take care of your comfort, even if it means turning off the news to relax in a bath, listening to soothing music with a cup of aromatic tea, or resting with your eyes closed.

- If you drink tea with caffeine throughout the day, you may wish to switch to tea with less or no caffeine starting after lunch.

- In your diary also write notes that help you check for stress and environmental factors. Write your feelings in your diary each day and trust the healing process with an open heart.

Complementary and folk favorites: Add a pinch of valerian root or damiana to Peaceful and Happy Tea, and take 2 to 4 kelp capsules before bedtime.

HOT FLASHES OR SWEATING

For many women, hot flashes are triggered by alcohol, sugar, food additives, artificial sweeteners, smoking, caffeine, and yang foods. For some of us, any hot beverage may start a hot flash. The reduction or elimination of these triggers can help considerably.

Vitamin E is known as "the menopause vitamin" because it has been used for estrogen replacement and has chemical activities that resemble estrogen. Taking vitamin E daily may reduce the frequency or severity of hot flashes and physiological symptoms of menopause. Five to ten almonds a day as a snack helps meet your vitamin E requirements. Many of my clients have reported positive results from eating these nuts.

Food therapy way: Follow cleansing plan A daily for two to three weeks and focus on cooling yin spices and medium to low glycemic index foods.

Specific prescription: A cup garbanzos daily and a cup of watermelon or juice before each meal; 2 to 3 tablespoons each (daily) of flaxseeds, fennel seeds, and barberries. Eat 3 to 4 ounces tofu, or 1 to 1½ cups garbanzos or hummus, or Sonia's Energizing Lentil Cereal (see chapter 4), ¼ cup cilantro (juiced), or a bunch of cilantro as a salad two to three times per week. Use sprouts of lentils, red clover, soybeans, and garbanzos in shakes, salads, sandwichs or sautés.

Avoid all triggers: Watch for spicy and hot yang foods, alcohol, and stressor foods. They can create a reaction of heat within your body. You can find clues to your personal reactions to foods in your food diary.

Tea way: Drink Healthy and Wise Tea (see chapter 5). Add a pinch of rose petals, damiana, and dandelion and red clover flowers to your green tea or mint tea.

Lifestyle: Wear light white cotton clothing to help your body breathe. Bed linens should also be made of pure cotton. Keep room temperatures cool. Bathe with rosewater, orange blossoms, or lavender extract. Use the scents of these flowers for aromatherapy or add their essential oils to massage oil.

Supplements: Vitamin E (400 to 800 IU daily), taken in the form of mixed tocopherols is suggested. Enzymes with multivitamins, calcium, zinc, magnesium, and Vitamin D. Progesterone cream works for some of my patients. Read the label carefully and choose the cream that has the highest percentage of progesterone or consult with your health professional.

Complementary and folk favorites: Black cohosh, chasteberry, yin chai hu (3 to 9 grams).

SYMPTOMS ASSOCIATED WITH MENOPAUSE

Follow the food wisdom pyramid. Focus on medium to low glycemic index foods. Be sure to record foods, mood swings, cravings, and symptoms, so you will know the effect of foods on your unique system.

Specific prescription: 1 cup garbanzos (may be roasted or in the form of hummus, or mixed with tofu) every day. Add 1 to 3 tablespoons each of rice bran and flaxseeds to your smoothie or cereal. Eat 2 to 4 cups of fruits and vegetables of all colors each day, and drink plenty of red-pigmented juice, such as grape, cranberry, or pomegranate.

Colors: All colors, with a focus on green, red, and purple.

Morning and snacking way: Sonia's Antioxidant Smoothie (see chapter 10) with roasted garbanzo powder or soy bran, berries, amaranth, millet, or quinoa and 1 teaspoon of crushed rose petals; roasted beets and yams; Boshki's Travel Snack (see chapter 6) with added dried berries, fennel seeds, cloves, anise, Roasted Garbanzos and Soybeans (see recipe in chapter 6), puffed brown rice, and almonds; a plate of basil, mint, sage, sprouted alfalfa, and grapes; brown rice cakes with seaweed and hummus.

Tea way: Healthy and Wise Tea (see chapter 5), Denna's Herbal Chai with soy or almond milk, Wise Flower Tea (see chapter 5), or other tea using damiana, licorice root, rose hips and petals, dandelion, fennel, anise, red clover leaves and flowers, dried berries, borage, alfalfa, sage, thyme, stevia, ginseng, or hibiscus. Add 1 teaspoon of powdered licorice root to your tea daily.

Lifestyle: Attach yourself to nature and detach yourself from negative energy. Practice qigong. Find a place, such as a retreat center, to go for a weekend, or make a space in your home a retreat place. Forgive yourself and others. Bring a symbol of peace, health, and good relationship whenever you retreat.

Supplements: Natural enzymes. Vitamins E (400 to 800 IU) and D, calcium, zinc, magnesium, and multivitamins (150 percent DV) without iron.

Complementary and folk favorites: Tincture or capsules of dong quai (angelica), black cohosh, chasteberry, vitex fruits, motherwort, bearberry, ginkgo biloba, unicorn root, or sarsaparilla.

OSTEOPOROSIS

Throughout our lives, our bodies replace cells, including bone cells. We now know scientifically how to prevent bone loss through plant foods. We know also that stressor foods lower absorption of calcium and accelerate bone loss. Although preventing osteoporosis is a process that should begin in childhood with healthy eating practices, you can still take positive steps to protect your bones at any time of life. The body's need for plant foods increases as hormonal levels (such as estrogen and progesterone) fall; sometimes by the time women reach their midthirties, their bodies may be replacing only about 1 percent of bone mass each year.

Food therapy way: Foods with boron and isoflavonoids increase your body's ability to hang on to estrogen and calcium.

Colors: Green, white, orange.

Specific prescription: Add 2 to 4 cups of combinations of these foods daily: plain yogurt; greens such as spinach or kale; amaranth toast spread with almond butter, avocado, and cheese (feta, low-fat Swiss, ricotta, cottage cheese); hummus; and 8 to 10 almonds per day. Occasionally make and eat soup stock from the bones of chicken or fish, or eat sardines including the bones or sautéed oysters. With all of these choices, it is easy to achieve your daily calcium needs. Taking enzymes and eating leafy greens will help you absorb calcium.

Avoid all triggers: Colored soda contain more phosphorous, which decreases calcium absorption, than clear soda. Too much animal protein and isolated protein such as soy may also decrease calcium absorption, as will smoking and overuse of alcohol.

Tea way: Drink fruit tea with culinary herbs, such as Healthy and Wise Tea, and green and black tea with berries, served with dried fruits.

Lifestyle: Sunshine gives you vitamin D, but avoid the heat of the day. Activity increases bone density, especially weight-bearing exercises such as lifting books and brisk walking with arm weights. Stretching while sitting on the floor is good for muscles and bones, as is applying pressure to acupressure points.

Supplements: To increase calcium absorption include enzymes, zinc, copper, vitamins D, K, B_6, and B_{12}, potassium, and fluoride.

Complementary and folk favorites: Dandelions and watercress may seem to be just weeds, but this ancient plant has been used for powerful remedies and delicious summer wine. The leaves are high in calcium, magnesium, and vitamin A and are delicious as additions to salads or steamed or sautéed.

YOUR SKIN

One reason many women take hormone replacement therapy is their belief that hormones will keep their skin from wrinkling. In fact, no proof exists that hormones affect skin in this way. Most aging of our skin comes not from lack of estrogen but by exposure to the sun and free radicals, and dehydration. The best way to prevent loss of moisture from the skin and help deter further skin aging is to wear a sunscreen with an SPF of 15 or 20.

If you spend a lot of time in the sun, it's important to wear a hat. Remember that too much exposure to the sun, especially around noontime, not only promotes wrinkles—it also causes skin cancer. Free radicals destroy collagen and elastin in skin in response to sun and oxidation. Smoking also increases your risk from the sun.

Food Wisdom for Protecting Your Skin

Nourishment for all skin problems starts internally. Many cultures believe a plant-based diet rich in essential fatty acids enhances the chemistry of skin.

Here are some tips:

Food therapy way: Adopt the eating plan for cleansing plan A for two weeks. Eat fruits and culinary herbs to get the benefit of antioxidants. These protect the skin and give you nutrient-rich blood throughout your body for longer cellular life.

- Eat cooling yin food plants like watermelon, watercress, cilantro, and arugula to help purify the blood.

- Eat a nutritious diet rich in vitamins. Include essential fatty acids from sources such as olive oil, nuts, and seeds such as flaxseeds and also sunflower seeds. Eat wheat germ, beans sprouts, almonds, and avocados, which are high in nutritious essential fatty acids and vitamin E. Some research shows that zinc and iodine also benefit the skin.

- Water, herbal tea, and a high-fiber diet hydrate the skin and help remove toxins from the body. Drink water frequently, all day long, and eat a lot of fruit. You will see the results.

Avoid all triggers: Cut stressor foods, high glycemic index foods, and avoid excessive alcohol. Although alcohol increases blood circulation, giving you a rosy glow, this effect is better obtained through exercise. Many people do not realize that drinking beer and other alcoholic beverages causes dehydration.

- Smoking Harms the Skin: Smoking leads to premature aging. It damages collagen and elastin and decreases blood flow to the skin. The importance of stopping smoking to improve your health cannot be overemphasized. While smoking may tranquilize the brain for about fifteen minutes after a cigarette, its long-term effects are disastrous.

Tea way: Healthy and Wise Tea, chamomile, lavender, black currant, berry, and borage teas are used by many cultures and help cleanse your system, facilitating good skin.

Complementary and folk favorites: For skin eruptions, acne, boils, eczema, and pimples, women of ancient Greek and Roman times, as well as women of the Middle East put fig juice and pulp on the skin for healing. You can try it.

INCONTINENCE

More than thirteen million women and men in the United States suffer from urinary incontinence. Incontinence can be caused by depression, emotional distress, urinary tract infections, inflammation, or the effects of medication. Weakness of the bladder is not a natural consequence of aging. Many people with incontinence feel that they never completely empty the bladder. Eat hormonally and practice Kegel exercises—contracting the pelvic muscles periodically while driving, exercising, or urinating. A major study shows a relationship between incontinence and weight gain, so eating patterns and food choices may be an issue (Lean 2000). For incontinence problems, cut alcohol, soda, coffee, black and green tea, and other stressor foods because they are diuretic. Herbal tea with no caffeine supports and nourishes the kidney and gallbladder.

URINARY TRACT INFECTIONS

Infections may be caused by bacteria from the colon entering the urinary tract. Use antibacterial foods such as yogurt, garlic, ginger, and yang spices. Eat more red-colored fruits and vegetables to keep your urine pH balanced to combat infections. Follow cleansing plan A with seeds in cranberry and pomegranate juice; alternate the juices each morning and drink lots of water with diverse seeds during the day. In studies, when women drank cranberry juice, they were 58 percent less likely to get urinary tract infections; if they already had an infection, they were able to heal 27 percent faster from the infection (Ingels 2002). These berries are available in capsules, but why not enjoy them more deliciously, in recipes and tea?

VAGINAL INFECTIONS & OTHER PROBLEMS

You can balance alkaline vaginal tissues, which can be susceptible to bacterial or yeast infections, by eating yogurt or yang foods. Prevent harmful conditions by using the cleansing way and by drinking plenty of water and tea. Lower your consumption of diuretic foods, such as alcohol and caffeine. Estrogen loss thins vaginal tissues, so keep your estrogen and progesterone balanced.

Take extra enzyme supplements, vitamin C, and yogurt mixed with dried mint 3 times daily.

Vaginal Dryness and Vaginitis (Vaginal Infections)

Vaginal dryness may be the result of hormone fluctuations or thyroid problems. Chronic vaginitis may be an immune imbalance, but it is often caused by yeast overgrowth and may lead to vaginal dryness and contribute to sexual discomfort. For vaginitis or vaginal dryness, eat hormonal foods (hummus, tofu, berries, yams, and sweet potatoes) and boron foods (grapes, raisins, and apples). Drinking more water or herbal tea may increase mucus throughout the body, including the vagina. Eat foods with essential fatty acids and vitamin E. Take enzyme supplements. Research has proven the health benefits of yogurt (Genet 1995). Eat 1 to 3 cups daily of yogurt with pinch of lactobacillus, ginger, mint, and garlic; include 1 to 3 cups of antioxidant foods (cranberry and pomegranate juice) in the cleansing way.

Estrogen and progesterone cream (4 to 7 percent) used externally or a lubricant such as vitamin E oil helps some women. Some cultures believe having more frequent sex and adding mistletoe to tea will help vaginal dryness.

Low Sex Desire

Eat hormonally and colorfully. Dancing, listening to music, reading a good book, drinking tea, meditation, exercise, and walking can all increase your sense of physical well-being, causing endorphins and serotonin to stimulate your libido. Around the world, women enjoy sexual relationships more after menopause because they no longer need to worry about pregnancy and childbearing. The herb damiana and red clover leaves and flowers in your tea may stimulate your sex drive. Damiana leaves, from a shrub that thrives in Mexico, have been a folk aphrodisiac for more than a century.

chapter 9

the joy of spices
& herbs

Art, dance, poems, food and cooking connects us together.
—Thich Nhat Hanh

to learn to put the food wisdom pyramid into action in your life and revolutionize your thinking about food and your health, start with the flavor of herbs and spices. Your body will thrive in health and beauty when spiced foods are added to your life. Some studies have suggested that the low incidence of cardiovascular disease in parts of Spain may be related to the Spanish love of the spice saffron. Some spices, like cardamom and ginger, can kill up to fifteen different harmful bacterial species (Sherman and Billings 1998).

Culinary herbs and spices have their own chapter in this book because they are very important for women in all their cellular, hormonal, and other bodily systems during all ages of their lives. Their value as nutrients is so misunderstood. More and more research shows the phytoestrogenic nature of herbs and spices and their role in boosting the immune system. Spices have never been a part of any food pyramid. They are primary in mine.

spices & herbs, blended into your life

Since the food wisdom pyramid is different from any other, let us think in a different way about spices and culinary herbs. Instead of thinking of them as a garnish or as ingredients that add flavor (which of course they do), thinks of them instead as a basic food need.

Of course, spices and herbs are blended into everything you eat with food wisdom recipes. Culinary herbs and spices interact with all the other pyramid foods. They permeate these foods with flavor. ❧

relearning the wisdom of herbs & spices

Herbs, and plants in general, where our phytoestrogens and antioxidants come from, are humankind's first medicine and their use as such has been prominent in all cultures throughout history. Most cultures have taken thousands of years to develop the use of herbs and other plants in healing practices, through trial and error. A quarter of the drugs we use come from plants. We now recognize that many herbs and spices have healing properties and are much safer compared to drugs when used properly. Comparisons made between treating conditions with a drug and treating with a Chinese herb formula showed the herbs stimulated the body to rid itself of the disturbing factor while the drug acted, but depressed the body (Dharmananda 1998).

HERBS FOR HORMONAL BALANCE

In my research with Dr. David Zava, we have found that many culinary herbs and spices contain progesterone or estrogen, the hormones that many menopausal women may lack, and this is just one example of their value.

Certain herbs and spices can help with PMS and pre- and post-menopausal symptoms. Many herbs contain substances that can help relieve or prevent imbalances in our metabolism.

UNDERSTANDING SAFE USAGE

We know spices protect us by killing harmful bacteria, so we must use them selectively to control their effectiveness, and to not overkill the bacteria in our bodies. A serious problem from use of herbs may arise when someone believes that just because herbs are natural, you can pop herbal pills like candy. An herb that has the ability to help heal also has the ability, if misused, to harm. Too much of any food can be very unhealthy, so before you start adding herbs and spices into your diet, you need to be informed.

Infants and nursing and pregnant mothers should use only the medicines and herbal products their nutritionists or doctors advise.

Herbal products should be used wisely, and it's important to become informed. The American Herbal Products Association has a consumer reference manual on six hundred herbs with directions for safe use. Go to www.ahpa.com to learn more. I buy herbs or supplements from well-known companies who offer organic products and products derived from whole foods, because they will usually take extra precautions on labeling and take responsibility for the way herbs are gathered and prepared. Use only the recommended dosage, and if you begin to experience unusual symptoms after adding a new herb to your diet, discontinue its use.

DISTINGUISHING HERBAL MEDICINES FROM CULINARY HERBS

In many cultures, herbs are divided into two categories: herbal medicines and culinary herbs. In the food wisdom pyramid, I recommend only culinary herbs, which can be used generously. These include parsley, cilantro, peppermint, spearmint, dill, and others. Culinary herbs make wonderful garnishes. They not only brighten up a plate but, when eaten after the meal, freshen your breath because they contain chlorophyll. Green herbs not only please your palate and senses but also cleanse your liver and spleen, promote healthy enzymes and good bacteria, help in the absorption and digestion of nutrients, strengthen your bone density, balance your blood oxygen level and your body's alkalinity, and provide nutrients. Parsley, for example, is rich in vitamins A and C. ❧

spice & herb tips

So what to eat and not to eat? Here are some recommendations.

SUGAR & SPICE

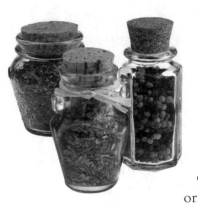

Contrary to what you have learned from childhood in old nursery rhymes, sugar and spice are not everything nice. Your spice can serve you well without so much added sugar! Spices and herbs do not have a glycemic index (see chapter 7) and may help balance insulin.

If you have a sweet tooth, instead of indulging it with sugar or artificial sweeteners, add spice. Spices in your foods and shakes will make you healthier and keep your taste buds happy. Add a pinch of licorice root (powdered or chopped) or cinnamon to baked apples, hot teas, ciders, and juices. Sprinkle nutmeg over applesauce or hot lemonade. Add cloves to chutney, relishes, and marinades. Other sweet spices you might experiment with are allspice and vanilla.

GARLIC FOR HIGH IMMUNITY

Another food wisdom choice for overall healing is garlic and its sister foods: onions, chives, leeks, shallots, and green onions. Whole books have been written about the antibiotic and cholesterol-lowering properties of garlic and its active ingredient, *allicin*. Most cultures have cooked with it in one form or another for thousands of years, and many recommend it for its antibacterial, antiviral, and antifungal properties. Ancient Greek and Roman physicians such as Hippocrates and Pliny the Elder recommended garlic to help with respiratory problems, to lose weight, to gain energy, and to treat many other conditions. Studies show that garlic can kill at least seventy-two infectious bacteria, including those that spread botulism, tuberculosis, dysentery, and diarrhea.

The green leaves of the garlic plant are great mixed with steamed rice or in soup. Garlic will help the good bacteria in your gut flourish while preventing colds and heart disease and alleviating yeast overgrowth.

If you're uncomfortable at work with garlic breath, eat garlic mostly on weekends or try this: after eating garlic, chew fresh parsley, cucumber, mint, or dried tea, or use any breath freshener and brush your teeth thoroughly. And remember, if you get everybody around you to enjoy garlic, no one will notice *your* breath.

If you don't like garlic, you can substitute shallots, onions, green onions, chives, and leeks in your recipes. Onions also exert positive effects on the body.

Garlic and onions go hand in hand in almost all my recipes. Sonia's Basic Onion Formula (see chapter 10) is pungent with garlic and excellent for flavoring meat when you want to use only a small amount of meat.

You can simply bake onions and whole garlic to spread on your bread like butter, or use garlic as a single herb for your meat, fish, and vegetable dishes. Have you ever tried garlic, herb, and yogurt sauce? Or garlic yogurt cheese? Or pickled garlic, aged for several years? See my Basic Onion Formula and Aged Garlic recipes in chapter 10.

TURMERIC: TODAY'S ANTIOXIDANT

Turmeric, a root of the ginger family, is a popular spice, and its phytoestrogenic and antioxidant properties are currently receiving a lot of medical research attention. The intense yellow-orange color of turmeric comes from the antioxidant curcumin and vitamin A. Scientists have documented turmeric as a natural anti-inflammatory substance with abilities to suppress the growth of the blood vessels that feed tumors (Nakamura et al. 1999).

Today turmeric is grown mainly in China, Indonesia, India, Iran, Haiti, and Jamaica, and is a major ingredient for making curry powder, mustard, and marinades for broiled chicken or fish, and is used in salads, sauces, and dressings. Try it in your eggs, in soups and stews, and with sauteed onions. See Sonia's Basic Onion Formula recipe in chapter 10. It gives a bright color, aroma, and distinct flavor to food.

CURRY: ANTIOXIDANT OF INDIA

Curry is the aroma of India's cuisine. The word *curry* refers to a blend of ground spices, including turmeric, fenugreek, cumin seed, coriander, and red or cayenne pepper. Some curries also contain allspice, cinnamon, cardamom, cloves, fennel, and other spices. Though still controversial, some experts believe that the carotene in curry may help prevent cancer.

In India, curries are used in hundreds of dishes made with fish, beans, mushrooms, meat, poultry, eggs, vegetables, and legumes. Curry dishes are usually served on rice, which absorbs the sauce.

GINGER: ANTIOXIDANT OF ASIA

For centuries, ginger was considered a medicine as well as a spice, and even today some cultures prescribe it as a digestive stimulant. The Chinese believed that fresh ginger would stimulate the stomach, much as pepper does. They made candied ginger as a dessert. Many Native American tribes used wild ginger medicinally. The Ojibwa Indians, for example, used a warm poultice of wild ginger to aid in healing arm fractures. My own flu- and cold-fighting soup recipe is filled with green onions, mushrooms, and ginger (see Immunity-Boosting Miso Soup in chapter 10).

Fresh ginger, sold as gingerroot, will keep for a week or so if refrigerated in paper wrap. (To store for about a year, peel the root, cut into half-inch slices, and immerse in dry sherry or rice vinegar; cover and refrigerate.) Fresh ginger—shredded, minced, sliced, or grated—can perk up soups and stews, marinades, stir-fried dishes, and salads. When added to cooking water, it spices up green beans, carrots, sweet potatoes, and winter squash. A few drops of ginger juice, pressed from the root, can flavor salad dressings. Boiling the root in water, or adding boiling water to ginger, makes a wonderful tea.

CHILE PEPPERS: FITNESS & METABOLISM

The chile is a tropical American plant from whose peppers we get cayenne and hot pepper sauce. Chili powder is a blend of dried chile peppers, ground with sweeter Mexican chiles, and sometimes cumin seed and oregano. Chili powder stimulates the lungs and helps with allergies and breathing problems.

Jean Carper (1988), in her book *The Food Pharmacy*, cites an Oxford Polytechnic study, which found that adding a few grams of hot chilie sauce and mustard to a meal increased participants' metabolic rate by up to 25 percent. I buy red crushed pepper and use it very successfully in soups, stews, omelets, and pilafs.

PEPPERCORNS: AIDING DIGESTION

Black pepper is one of the most popular spices in the world. It comes as whole peppercorns, cracked, or ground. Research shows that in cultures where people consume a lot of pepper, there are fewer stomach problems. One reason is that pepper stimulates the membranes of the mouth and stomach wall, making the muscles stronger. Pepper produces an increase in stomach acids, which helps aid digestion. Pepper can be used on almost any food—eggs, meat, poultry, salads, and vegetables— because it doesn't mask the flavor of food but adds pungency and zest.

CUMIN, FENNEL, GINGER, LICORICE, THYME, & ROSEMARY: SPICES FOR DIGESTION

Spices such as fennel, licorice, ginger, thyme, and rosemary are used in various cultures after meals to comfort and aid digestion and harmonize the hormones, and much is being learned in Western culture about their properties and their combination with seeds, fruits, vegetables, and high-fiber foods. Licorice can be bought (powdered, crushed, or dried) in the herbs and seasoning section of health food stores or major grocery stores. Try my recipes throughout the book that use these great spice flavors. You can only enhance your health.

SUMAC, SAGE, SEAWEED: FOODS FOR THE HEART

Sumac, sage, and seaweed may benefit your heart. The American Heart Association is conducting extensive research on these spices as healthy alternatives to salt.

There could be an entire book on sage, which is an appetite stimulant, helping you appreciate all other foods. For eating hormonally, add sage to your tea, soup, stew, and snacks. Put it on cheese, yogurt, and sandwiches. Sasha's Mood Burritos (see chapter 10) use seaweed instead of salt to build bone.

FRESH DILL & DILL SEEDS FOR LOWERING CHOLESTEROL

I am working on study on the use of fresh dill in reducing cholesterol. Although we are still working on the study, it seems to lower cholesterol 60 percent, with an increase of the "good" cholesterol (HDL). Regardless of what the study eventually determines about cholesterol, dill is nutritious and benefits your body. Dill is delicious as a salad or mixed with cucumber and yogurt. You can add a cup of dill or a tablespoon of dill seeds to rice, frozen soybeans, potatoes, stews, and other recipes. You can support your cleansing day with dill, along with other culinary herbs and spices.

VINEGAR FOR DIGESTION

Vinegar is a way to add flavor, and some ethnic groups consider it a spice, though it is not from a spice plant, but is made from apples, rice, or grapes. Judicious use of vinegar helps keep the body's alkalinity and acidity balanced for healthy enzymes. Some people drink a glass of warm water and vinegar (5 percent apple cider) before eating or before beginning a cleansing program. Lemon and lime have similar uses. How your body's digestion will benefit from vinegar, lime, and lemon depends on your body's acidity and alkalinity. Balsamic vinegar makes a tasty salad dressing. Combine it with one or two drops of oil, or skip the oil altogether. Seasoned rice vinegar has a sweet taste and is also excellent on salad. ❧

LEMON SPICES UP YOUR FOOD, PEEL & ALL

Lemons are used mostly for fish, stews, tea, and jam. Lemon zest, the outer rind of the fruit, can be grated to spice up salads, breads, marinades, and sauces for veal, chicken, lamb, and fish. In Middle Eastern and Mediterranean cultures, dried lemon is used instead of salt. Try it! Use fresh lemon and lime with olive oil, spices, and herbs (dill, mint, oregano, pepper) as a dressing for fish. Eating the white part of citrus fruits for digestion is a Middle Eastern custom and research is showing this part of citrus fruits to be high in antioxidants. ❧

zoe's story

Zoe was a Buddhist practicing Zen meditation and had high spiritual values. She needed help because of very bad joint pain, low energy, fatigue, hot flashes, and asthma. She was also concerned about surgery scheduled for one knee.

It was a very hard case for me because Zoe already seemed to be doing everything right with her lifestyle and vegetarian diet. She was eating a very plain, fresh, whole-foods diet, but it was completely lacking in spices and what I consider essential herbs, such as turmeric and mint. The problem was she was not getting enough magnesium, enzymes. zinc, folic acid, selenium, chromium, and vitamins E and D.

Along with adding turmeric to her diet, two tablespoons every day to use in recipes, I asked her to drink one tablespoon of turmeric mixed with one tablespoon of miso paste stirred in 2 tablespoons of apple cider vinegar and a cup of warm water. She followed the tea way and used lots of healthy snacks, eating small amounts every two hours.

I also advised her to put a paste of garbanzo flour, flaxseed oil, turmeric, and peppermint on grape leaves under her knee bandage. She slept with this on at night and changed the leaves frequently during the day. She also was taking a capsule of turmeric per meal.

Her body's yin and yang and acidity and alkalinity were unbalanced, so I added hot properties to her food plan: more cinnamon, nutmeg, and cayenne pepper to help her blood circulate and heat her joints.

Within five weeks her symptoms had largely gone away. Her hot flashes disappeared, and she had an increase in energy; her pain lessened, the inflammation disappeared, and she decided not to have surgery. At our annual visit, I was glad to find that she was doing a lot of exercise, swimming, and was happy playing tennis without any pain. She had lost some weight, which relieved the pressure on her joints. ✄

the art of flavoring with herbs & spices

Flavoring with herbs and spices is a creative adventure, and success is measured entirely by your own tastes. Here are some time-honored combinations, to increase your knowledge and spark your inventiveness.

- tofu: pomegranate paste, hoisin sauce or prune paste, saffron with lemon, or soy sauce with ginger and vinegar

- hummus: turmeric, curry, saffron, parsley, cayenne pepper, basil, or lemon and olive oil

- beef: bay leaf, chervil, tarragon, marjoram, parsley, savory, rosemary, garlic, turmeric, chiles, lemon or lime juice, or green onions

- cheese: basil, chervil, chives, curry, dill, fennel, garlic, mint, oregano, parsley, sage, or thyme

- fish: chervil, dill, fennel, tarragon, garlic, parsley, thyme, basil, chiles, yogurt with saffron, lemon or lime juice, or bay leaf

- fruit: seeds and nuts, anise, cinnamon, coriander, cloves, ginger, mint, nutmeg, or cardamom

- lamb: garlic cloves, mint, clover seeds, marjoram, oregano, rosemary, thyme, turmeric, baby onions, or saffron

- poultry: garlic, oregano, rosemary, savory, turmeric, saffron, sage, onion, parsley, marjoram, or ginger

- salads: basil, chives, tarragon, garlic, parsley, sorrel, pepper, cinnamon, dill, celery seeds, green onions, mint, pepper, or cumin; herb vinegars are also useful flavorings

- vegetables: basil, chervil, chives, parsley, dill, tarragon, marjoram, mint, pepper, thyme, garlic, green onions, celery seeds, or savory

HERB BLENDS

Some foods have an affinity with certain flavorings. Knowing that the results will always be good, you can have these blends on hand as quick, simple flavorings:

- barbecue blend: cumin, garlic, hot pepper, oregano, and cloves

- egg herbs: basil, dill weed, chiles, chives, and parsley (add fresh green onion and tomatoes when cooking)

- Italian blend: basil, marjoram, oregano, rosemary, sage, savory, thyme, and chives

- tomato sauce herbs: basil, bay leaf, marjoram, oregano, parsley, and chiles

Pungent Salt Substitute

1 tablespoon dried basil
1 teaspoon each celery seeds, rosemary, coriander seeds, dried savory, cumin seeds, dried sage, dried marjoram, and dried lime (or citric accid crystals)
2 teaspoons sumac powder

Mix well, and then powder with a mortar and pestle.

SALT SUBSTITUTES

Salt is such an easy flavoring to use—and abuse. Here is an herb blend substitute that you can make up and keep handy, perhaps stored in a commercial herb bottle. Sumac can be purchased from Middle Eastern markets. You can find citric acid crystals in health food stores. Whatever you do, avoid commercial salt substitutes unless you have permission from your doctor to use them.

chapter 10

recipes for balanced hormones

*The journey of a thousand miles
begins with a single step.*
—Lao Tze

my original, easy-to-use recipes provide abundance, resources, and hormonal foods for women who want to cook foods rich in the ingredients of the food wisdom pyramid, inspired by a variety of cultures. Flavorful and colorful recipes integrate the food wisdom ways with foods rich in phytoestrogens, essential fatty acids, protein, fiber, and antioxidants. These recipes merge scientific studies with practicality and the wisdom behind healing with foods.

These recipes are designed for maximum flavor, minimal calories, yang-yin balance, and increased enzymes for good digestion. Common ingredients are used in new combinations and with flavors that you will find enticingly exotic, with many available substitutions and options. ❧

the basics

Sonia's Basic Onion Formula

MAKES 2 CUPS

A versatile, flavorful formula for a soup, stew, or seasoning base for vegetables, grains, and herbs. This recipe is easy and fast. I use it as a base for most of my recipes for stew, chiles, or soup, and combine it with pasta and vegetables to serve with a green salad for a quick dinner. Keep this on hand to use any time. If you are making it to store in the refrigerator or freezer, triple the recipe. The seasoning base can be stored in the refrigerator up to one month or in the freezer for four months. You can use 2 tablespoons at a time for a recipe base.

> **2 medium red or white onions, chopped**
> **2 tablespoons olive oil, or as desired**
> **Pinch of salt**
> **2 to 4 cloves garlic, chopped or minced, or I teaspoon garlic powder (optional)**
> **I to 3 teaspoons turmeric**

Place the onions and olive oil in a large, heavy saucepan over medium-high heat. Stiring constantly, add the salt and let the onions become translucent and then caramelize, about 5 minutes.

When the onions are turning golden brown, turn the heat to medium and add the garlic and turmeric. Continue cooking about 2 minutes.

Marinated Tofu

MAKES 2¾ CUPS

You can use marinated tofu as a substitute for meat in any meal. Add it to dishes of rice or beans.

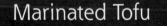

> **I pound tofu, cut in 3- to 4-inch squares**
> **½ cup balsamic or seasoned rice vinegar or orange or pomegranate juice**
> **2 tablespoons toasted sesame oil**
> **I teaspoon each chopped ginger, garlic, and cumin seeds**

Drain the tofu and press it to remove more liquid.

Add the remaining ingredients to the tofu. Mix thoroughly and refrigerate for at least 20 minutes so the tofu can absorb the flavors.

MAKES 4 SERVINGS

These burritos provide lots of energy through the beans. No one misses cheese if you add avocado to a burrito. My client Sasha is the one who first told me that she put dried seaweed, a good mood booster, on burritos, and so I've named this recipe in her honor.

1 16-ounce can vegetarian refried beans, red beans, or garbanzo beans

8 tortillas (corn, spinach, or flour)

2 sheets of seaweed

2 Anaheim chiles, chopped

6 green onions, chopped (including green part)

½ cup salsa, fresh or from a jar

1 cup fresh cilantro

2 cups chopped arugula or lettuce (optional)

1 tablespoon sour cream (optional)

2 ripe avocados, divided into quarters

8 ripe olives (optional)

Heat the beans in saucepan or microwave.

Warm the tortillas in a warm oven or skillet.

Roast the seaweed on the burner of a stove for a few seconds, but don't burn it!

Spoon the warmed beans on to the tortilla and top with the seaweed, chiles, onions, salsa, and cilantro. If desired, top with arugula and sour cream. Put one-quarter of an avocado and 2 olives on each burrito, fold the tortillas to enclose the filling, and enjoy!

Variations: *Instead of red beans or garbanzo beans, use canned black beans blended with 2 or 3 cloves of garlic and cilantro. You can also use a combination of black and pinto beans. Add roasted chicken, turkey, tuna, or chopped hard-cooked egg whites for more tryptophan.*

Persian Ab-Gosht
(Lamb Stew)

MAKES 4 SERVINGS

This is easy, aromatic, filling, and balanced, nourishing all your senses. It brings family and friends together. This is Persian culture's signature dish.

I cup each garbanzo beans and white flat beans (soaked together overnight)

I pound lamb with bone (leg or lamb chop)

2 cups chopped eggplant

4 to 6 medium potatoes, whole or chopped

4 to 6 medium tomatoes, chopped

I large onion, chopped

4 to 6 cloves garlic

I tablespoon each (or to taste) turmeric, sea salt, crushed red or black pepper, and cinnamon

Juice of I lime

Cinnamon, for garnish

Drain the soaked beans.

Put all the ingredients except the lime juice and cinnamon in a big pot with 4 quarts of water. Cook over medium heat until the beans are tender, about 2 hours. Add more water if the stew becomes dry.

Season with the lime juice. Remove all the broth you can with a ladle or soup spoon and reserve in a bowl.

Remove the lamb bone and cut the meat from the bone.

Mash or blend the cooked beans, vegetables, and meat together to make a consistency like stuffing or mashed potatoes. Add broth as needed to reach the desired consistency. Scoop this mixture into serving dishes. Sprinkle each with cinnamon.

Serve with bread and fresh mint, basil, pickles, or yogurt. Serve the broth as a clear soup or drink it.

Variations: *Meatless Ab-Gosht, exclude the meat and double the eggplant. For arthritis, increase the turmeric to ¼ cup, add 2 cups chopped fresh parsley, and omit the eggplant and tomatoes.*

Russian Caviar Surprise

MAKES 4 SERVINGS

The surprise is it's eggplant! This creamy dish, while providing many nutrients, will surprise even those who don't like eggplant because it has the consistency of meat. In the Mediterranean, women slice eggplant, sprinkle it with salt (to remove the bitter flavor), and leave it on platters on the roof or balconies to sun dry, creating a chewy, delicious snack full of the sun's energy. You can cook the pulp and freeze it for later. If you like spicy food, add a dash of cayenne pepper.

> **4 medium eggplants**
> **2 to 4 tablespoons olive oil**
> **4 cloves garlic, minced**
> **⅔ cup minced green onions**
> **¼ cup chopped fresh dill, loosely packed, or**
> **1 tablespoon dried**
> **2 tablespoons poppy seeds**
> **1½ cups plain yogurt cheese (or plain yogurt, drained of juice)**
> **Salt and pepper**
> **8 kalamata or ripe green olives, for garnish**
> **2 tablespoons roasted sesame seeds or flaxseeds, for garnish**

Preheat the oven to 400°F.

Cut the eggplants in half lengthwise, and salt and brush the cut part with oil. Bake for 20 to 40 minutes or until very soft.

Remove the pulp from the baked eggplants and discard the skin. Mix in the garlic, green onions, dill, poppy seeds, and yogurt cheese, and season with pepper. Garnish with olives and seeds and serve with crackers, toasted pita, or vegetables for dipping, or serve in a sandwich.

Variations: *Substitute 2 medium tomatoes, chopped, for the yogurt cheese. Substitute 1 cup silky tofu and 2 tablespoons lemon juice or ½ cup tahini for the yogurt cheese. Grill the eggplant on a charcoal grill instead of baking. This adds a smoky flavor and is great during the summer barbecue season when eggplants are plentiful. For a party, cut the top off a large round of sourdough bread, scoop out some of the bread (save for another use). Fill the round with the eggplant caviar and garnish as above.*

Gaemi Girl's Spaghetti

MAKES 8 SERVINGS

My daughter-in-law doesn't cook much, but this dish helped her discover the joy and ease of good food. Now, she proudly serves it to family and friends, bringing it to potlucks and passing out the recipe. Best of all, it makes enough sauce to freeze portions for future meals. The tortillas in the bottom of the pan create a crusty, crunchy delight.

2 medium onions, diced
2 to 4 cloves garlic, minced, or 1 teaspoon garlic powder
2 tablespoons olive oil
1 tablespoon turmeric
1 pound ground beef or ground turkey or firm tofu (diced)
1 teaspoon cinnamon
½ cup fresh oregano or basil, chopped, or 1 tablespoon dried
1 16-ounce can kidney beans (drained)
1 16-ounce can chopped tomatoes or 5 to 8 diced fresh tomatoes
Salt and pepper
1 carrot, shredded
3 small zucchini squash, sliced
8 to 10 small mushrooms, sliced or cut into chunks
16 ounces spaghetti
2 flour tortillas
1 cup grated sharp cheddar or Jack cheese, or crumbled feta cheese (optional)
Crumbled feta, for garnish (optional)
A few olives, for garnish

Sauté the onions and garlic in the olive oil over medium heat in a large Dutch oven or other heavy, large pan. When the onion is clear and beginning to brown, add the turmeric and stir until the onion is evenly coated and yellow.

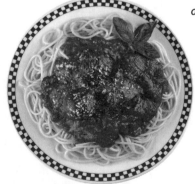

Add the ground beef (or turkey or tofu) and brown. Add the cinnamon, oregano or basil, kidney beans, and tomatoes. Mix well. Add salt and pepper to taste and simmer uncovered for 10 minutes. Add the carrot, zucchini, and mushrooms. Cover and simmer on low heat, stirring occasionally, for 10 to 15 minutes.

Preheat the oven to 450°F. Cook the spaghetti according to package directions in boiling, salted water with a splash of olive oil. Drain and rinse.

Slightly coat the bottom of a large ovenproof casserole or Dutch oven with olive oil. Layer the tortillas in the bottom of the pan. Mix a small amount of the spaghetti with some sauce and layer it on top of the tortilla layer. Add a layer of cheese if you are using it. Alternate layers

of spaghetti, sauce, and cheese until all the ingredients have been used. End with a
layer of sauce.

Cover and cook on the bottom shelf of the oven for 25 minutes. Remove from the oven
and carefully remove the pasta and put it on a large serving dish. (A spatula works
well for this.)

The tortilla layer will still be in the pan. Remove it, break into medium pieces, and serve
on a separate plate as an appetizer.

Garnish with crumbled feta and olives.

Variations: For serving in a hurry, toss the cooked spaghetti and sauce together, top with feta and
olives, and serve. Substitute 16 ounces frozen spinach (or 3 bunches fresh) for the zucchini. Serve
with persian cold soup, a plate of fresh herbs, cucumber, and fresh tomato, or yogurt mixed with
cucumber and dried mint.

Noble High-Energy Garbanzo Pilaf

MAKES 4 TO 6 SERVINGS

For this recipe, I gave garbanzo beans the title of noble food, because they are one of the
strongest and purest energy-creating foods and they boost the hormonal qualities women
need to protect their bodies. This recipe makes a complete meal and the spices make the
food rich with flavor and color to appeal to your sensuous side.

- **2 medium onions, minced**
- **2 to 4 tablespoons olive oil**
- **2 to 4 cloves garlic, minced**
- **I tablespoon sliced ginger**
- **I teaspoon each turmeric, cumin seeds, cinnamon, and saffron powder (optional)**
- **2 medium red bell peppers, minced**
- **2 cups each garbanzo beans (cooked or canned and drained), uncooked long-grain brown rice, firm tofu (diced), and tomatoes (minced)**
- **4 cups warm water or broth (vegetable, chicken, or miso)**
- **Salt and pepper**
- **Fresh mint or basil sprigs, for garnish**

Preheat the oven to 375°F.

In a large pot, sauté the onions and garlic in the oil for 5 minutes.

Add all the remaining ingredients except the garnish and stir to blend flavors.

Place the mixture in a large, shallow baking dish, cover, and bake for 45 to 50 minutes,
or until the rice is tender.

Remove the lid, fluff the pilaf with two forks, and top with the garnish before serving.

Variations: Substitute 2 cups of couscous, amaranth, bulgur, quinoa, or triticale for the rice (rice
cooking times may vary). Substitute green soybeans or diced green beans for the garbanzos. Serve
with yogurt, fresh green herbs such as basil and mint, and green onions.

Koosha's Green Herb Frittata

This is a bone food because of the greens and a cleansing food because it nourishes the liver. The protein feeds the muscles and other body systems. It's an excellent source of antioxidants. Serve it over rice with fish or use it in sandwiches with pickles. Yogurt, rice, and bread complement this dish nicely.

4 eggs

3 egg whites (optional)

3 cups chopped parsley

3 cups cilantro leaves

1 cup chopped spinach leaves

3 cups green onions, finely minced

2 teaspoons turmeric

Pinch of cinnamon

2 tablespoons all-purpose flour

Salt and pepper

3 tablespoons olive oil

½ cup chopped walnuts or almonds, for garnish

½ cup dried berries, for garnish

Preheat the oven to 350°F.

Beat the eggs and egg whites in a large mixing bowl. Stir in the parsley, cilantro, spinach, green onions, turmeric, cinnamon, flour, and salt and pepper to taste.

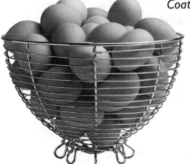

Coat a 14-inch ovenproof pan with the olive oil. Heat the pan in the oven for 5 minutes. Remove the pan from the oven and add the egg mixture. Cover with foil. Bake for 20 minutes. Remove the pan from the oven and uncover. Place under the broiler to brown the top, 5 to 15 minutes more, then remove from the oven and let set for about 10 minutes. Cut into slices and garnish each piece with the nuts and dried berries. Serve with fish and herbed rice.

Variation: *Heat some oil in a pan, and after step 2, ladle the mixture into the pan to make patties. Brown on both sides.*

morning way recipes

Sonia's Antioxidant Smoothie

MAKES I SMOOTHIE
(CAN BE MADE AND REFRIGERATED FOR 3 TO 4 DAYS)

Morning smoothies are a phytohormonal way to start the day, especially if you don't eat a balanced meal or are not accustomed to eating in the morning. Blended smoothies are preferable to juice, as they use the entire fruit and vegetable, including seeds, skin, and pulp, which are rich in phytohormones and fiber.

I hard-boiled egg, or 2 coddled egg whites (see directions below), or ½ cup egg substitute, or 2 teaspoons dried egg powder, or 2 tablespoons soy or roasted garbanzo flour

¼ cup soft tofu or ½ cup plain yogurt (or soy milk, almond milk, or a combination)

2 tablespoons rice bran

I to 3 tablespoons ground flaxseeds

I teaspoon honey (optional)

¼ cup frozen orange juice concentrate or raisins (optional)

Pinch of nutmeg, cardamom, ginger, or rose hips

I cup fresh, frozen, or dried berries of your choice (no strawberries)

Fresh mint sprig, cinnamon stick, or pinch of chocolate, for garnish

I cup unsweetened cranberry or pomegranate juice

Combine all the ingredients except the garnish and blend for 3 minutes in a blender. Serve immediately. Refrigerate any unused portion for future snacks or meals. Add more juice or water as needed.

Variations: *If you are using juice, add juice to smoothie to match specific fruit chosen (pear with pear juice, for example). To feed neurotransmitters (to balance mood), add I to 2 tablespoons of pumpkin seeds, kelp, or seaweed.*

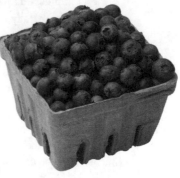

To coddle eggs: *Coddle whole eggs in their shells by placing them in boiling water for 3 minutes. Peel or crack the eggs and add to the smoothie. You can cook several eggs at once and store them in the refrigerator for up to one week.*

Colorful Antioxidant Smoothie

MAKES 2 SERVINGS

This is a variation on the basic smoothie recipe with emphasis in color. You can use yogurt, almond, walnut, tahini, or tofu, so it works for vegans, too. Make enough for a week, and freeze the base to use each morning with added fruits. Use the following colors depending on any symptoms you are experiencing, or for preventing health problems:

Colors for organs

Orange, yellow, and golden **for stomach and spleen: cantaloupe, mango, persimmon, all citrus fruits, carrots, banana, papaya, ginger.**

Green **to feed liver and pancreas: Broccoli, kale, arugula, spinach, celery, bok choy, chard, herbs (dill, cilantro, parsley, mint), watercress, assorted lettuce, seaweed, kiwi, green apples, green tea, green grapes**

Red and rose **to feed heart and hormones: Beets, strawberries, red grapes, cranberries, cherries, pomegranates, rose petals, peach, apricot**

Black **to feed kidney: black cherries, blackberries, black sesame seeds, cardamom seeds**

Purple **to feed moods: purple grapes, borage, lavender flowers, eggplant**

White **to feed lungs and colon: pears, turnips, potatoes, garlic, onion**

> **Ingredients:**
> ¼ **cup soft tofu or** ¼ **cup plain yogurt (or a combination)**
> **2 tablespoons soy flour or roasted garbanzo flour**
> **1 to 2 tablespoons oat bran, rice bran, or pysillim seeds (optional)**
> **1 to 2 tablespoon flax seeds or almond, or any nuts, seeds, or oil you fee you need therapeutically**
> **1 handful raisins, or** ½ **teaspoon honey (optional)**
> **2 to 3 ice cubes crushed, or your choice of flavored frozen yogurt, as desired**
> **1 cup fresh or frozen berries or watermelon**
> **fresh mint sprig, cinnamon stick, or nutmeg for garnish**

Combine all ingredients and blend for 3 minutes in a blender.

Garnish with berries and/or fresh mint.

If you are using juice, add juice to shake to match specific fruit chosen, such as juice of the berries you are using, or pomegranate or beets and their juice.

Variation: *Add one or more of these fruits and vegetables to the basic shake and blend for an additional 10 to 15 seconds: you may choose a color or mix and match different colors for depending on your needs:*

¼ cup strawberries, fresh or frozen; ¼ cup diced pineapple; ¼ banana with 2 drops vanilla and dash of cardamom; ¼ cup diced papaya; 1 small orange, diced and seeds removed; ¼ cup fresh or canned peaches, chopped; half medium apple, diced and 2 drops

Mediterranean Veggie Omelet

MAKES 4 SERVINGS

The ingredients in this colorful and tasty omelet are mixed right into the eggs, so prepara-tion is fast and easy, but your guests will rave about the flavors and your skills.

> **1 medium red onion, chopped**
> **2 cloves garlic, minced**
> **2 tablespoons oil**
> **1 cup sliced shitake mushrooms**
> **1 medium zucchini, chopped**
> **3 large tomatoes, chopped**
> **4 to 6 eggs**
> **½ cup olives, chopped**
> **3 to 4 ounces feta cheese, cubed**
> **1 cup grated part-skim mozzarella (optional)**
> **3 tablespoons fresh sage, basil, or thyme, minced, or ½ teaspoon dried**
> **herbs (optional)**

Sauté the onion and garlic in the oil in large skillet over medium heat. Add the mushrooms and zucchini, and cook for 2 minutes. Turn off the heat, add the tomatoes, and mix well. If you are making half the recipe, refrigerate half of these vegetables at this stage and use tomorrow.

Lightly beat the eggs and add, along with the olives, cheeses, and herbs, to the vegetable mixture. Cook over medium heat for 6 to 8 minutes.

Serve with toasted pita bread with fresh mint or with brown rice or pasta.

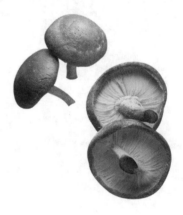

Variation: *Substitute diced broccoli, sprouted garbanzos, green soybeans, cucumber, eggplant, or asparagus for the zucchini.*

salads & greens

Happy Heart Red Beet Salad

MAKES 4 SERVINGS

Beets are heart food to people in the Middle East and are good for morning cleansing and strengthening the heart. The dark pigmentation indicates the presence of helpful antioxidants; beets are high in vitamin D, boron, folic acid and B complex vitamins, and fiber. The red turns the pasta a lovely shade of pink. If you prefer your pasta white, simply add the beets at the end, using them as a garnish.

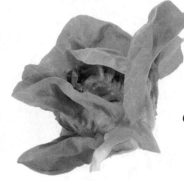

3 cups cooked pasta (shells, rigatoni, or wagon wheels)
3 cups cooked or canned beets, chopped
3 tablespoons poppy seeds (optional), plus extra for garnish
2 to 4 hard-boiled eggs, peeled and diced
2 tablespoons olive oil or mayonnaise
Juice of 2 lemons
Salt and pepper
Mixed salad greens

Combine all the ingredients except the greens, and mix well. Chill 10 to 20 minutes. Serve over the greens and garnish with poppy seeds.

Variations: Add ¼ cup plain yogurt. Substitute 2 tablespoons chopped walnuts for the poppy seeds. Add 1 cup sliced fennel root.

Berry Colorful Summer Salad

MAKES 4 TO 6 SERVINGS AS A SIDE DISH

Berries are nature's gift for women to help balance their hormones. High antioxidants, amazingly sweet and savory flavors, vivid colors, and crunch make this a great summertime salad.

> **I tablespoon olive oil**
> **2 cups French-cut green beans**
> **I large red bell pepper, finely chopped**
> **½ cup each fresh berries, slivered almonds, and pineapple juice**
> **I teaspoon each dill seeds and orange zest**
> **Salt and pepper**

Heat a large skillet or wok over medium heat. Add the oil, beans, bell pepper, berries, and almonds and cook for about 2 minutes, just until the beans are heated through.

Remove from the heat and add the pineapple juice, dill seeds, and orange zest. Combine thoroughly and season with salt and pepper.

Serve hot, or refrigerate and serve cold as a side salad. Alternatively, serve over basmati rice or soba noodles for a complete meal.

Variation: *Use 16-ounces of frozen green soybeans instead of green beans.*

Sautéed Leafy Greens

MAKES 5 CUPS

If you like to have delicious greens and culinary herbs, which are excellent for bone building, try this formula. Kale and yogurt are both bone foods and also good for relaxation. Sautéed kale makes a complete meal, or you can serve it as a side dish. It also makes a great dip for crisp wheat crackers and vegetables.

> **2 bunches or 5 cups kale or spinach (break the leaves from the stems and chop each separately)**
> **2 tablespoons Sonia's Basic Onion Formula (see recipe at the beginning of this chapter)**
> **2 cups low-fat yogurt**
> **½ cup chopped walnuts**
> **Pinch each of cinnamon, black pepper or cayenne, and sea salt**
> **I teaspoon chopped fresh ginger**
> **Toasted walnuts, for garnish**

Over medium heat sauté the greens for 3 to 5 minutes.

Add the onion base to the greens, cover, and steam over medium heat for 3 to 5 minutes. Remove from the heat, mix in the remaining ingredients except the garnish, and adjust seasonings to taste. Garnish with toasted walnuts and serve.

Variation: *Use greens such as spinach, chard, dandelion, purslane, and mustard greens instead of or in combination with the kale.*

Hearty Lentil-Rice Yin-Yang Balancing Salad

MAKES 4 TO 6 SERVINGS

The combination of ingredients in this salad may help balance your body's acidity and alkalinity. It can be made ahead and frozen, but omit the vinegar until you are ready to serve it.

3 cups cooked lentils

I cup cooked brown rice

I cup feta cheese or diced tofu (optional)

2 to 4 cloves garlic, minced

I small red onion, chopped

I small jalapeño pepper, seeded and minced (optional)

2 tablespoons balsamic or seasoned rice vinegar

2 tablespoons olive or sesame oil

¼ cup chopped olives (optional)

I cup chopped cilantro

Sea salt and pepper

Parsley sprigs, for garnish

Combine all the ingredients and mix well. Season with salt and pepper to taste and garnish with the parsley.

__Variations:__ Omit the rice, jalapeño, and cilantro, and add 2 cups of chopped fresh parsley. Substitute mung beans, black beans, or garbanzos for the lentils. Substitute bulgur wheat for all or part of the rice.

soups

MAKES 4 SERVINGS

This sweet and sour, refreshing, creamy-tasting soup makes a great appetizer or entrée and balances an overload of heat in your system, especially in summer. The flecks of fruit and green onion make it beautiful. This dish is good for building bones and calming the neurotransmitters.

4 cups low-fat plain yogurt (with live cultures)

2 cups peeled and diced or grated cucumber

½ cup each minced green onions, fresh mint, and dill (or 1 tablespoon each dried)

1 medium apple with skin, minced or grated (optional)

½ cup each raisins and roasted walnuts or pumpkin seeds

2 to 3 cloves garlic or 1 clove elephant garlic, minced

1 tablespoon dried rose petals (optional)

Salt and freshly ground pepper

Fresh herbs, such as dill or mint, or edible flowers, such as nasturtium, for garnish

Combine ingredients in the order listed.

Mix well and season with salt and pepper to taste. Refrigerate.

Just before serving, add cold water to adjust consistency. Serve with whole wheat bread, crackers, or pita bread. Crumble toasted bread or tortillas into the soup just before serving.

Variations: Add 2 hard-boiled chopped eggs for extra protein. Add flaxseeds for essential fatty acids. Add ¼ cup chopped shitake mushrooms and 2 tablespoons chopped fresh seaweed for added nutrients. Add 1 tablespoon dried green tea leaves and/or 1 teaspoon chopped fresh mint leaves.

Immunity-Boosting Miso Soup

MAKES 4 SERVINGS

Sip this soup before and throughout cold, flu, and allergy seasons to cleanse your body, rebuild your immune system, and help prevent illness.

2 tablespoons organic miso dissolved in 4 cups of water
1 cup shiitake mushrooms or any other mushrooms, chopped
1 bunch green onions, chopped (including green part)
1 tablespoon fresh ginger, shredded or chopped
1 teaspoon turmeric
½ teaspoon cayenne pepper, or to taste
1 tablespoon lemon juice or apple cider vinegar

Mix all the ingredients together and simmer for 10 minutes. Sip throughout the day.

Variations: This soup can be used as the base for vegetable soup. Add chopped carrots, green beans, zucchini, broccoli, kale, or Swiss chard. Serve with a dollop of yogurt and ground sesame seeds on top for extra protein.

Friendly Bacteria Ginger Soup

MAKES 4 SERVINGS

A warm hot soup to nourish your digestive system and to provide an environment for healthy, healing bacteria.

1 cup Sonia's Basic Onion Formula
1 teaspoon each ginger (powdered or finely chopped root), ground dried mint, dill
2 cups plain yogurt
1 cup garbanzo beans (canned or cooked and drained)

Put Sonia's Basic Onion Formula in a large pot
Dilute the yogurt with 5 cups of warm water and add to the pot with the onion and seasonings. Bring to just below boil over medium heat (don't allow yogurt to boil), stirring.
Add the garbanzo beans, dill, mint, and ginger and let simmer for 15 minutes.

Variations: Substitute canned soybeans or black-eyes peas for the garbanzo beans; Add ½ cup of cooked amaranth for extra protein and thickness.

MAKES 4 SERVINGS

This is a favorite for pungent taste and silky texture. Just sipping it gives a feeling of healing and comfort, especially on cleansing days. Poppy seeds sprinkled on this soup add a treat for the eyes as well as extra antioxidants and good fat.

- **1 cup Sonia's Basic Onion Formula**
- **1 package (16 ounces) frozen green peas or sweet green soybeans**
- **1 jalapeño chile, chopped**
- **2 cups fresh or frozen corn**
- **2 bunches fresh cilantro, thoroughly rinsed**
- **1 lb. tomatillos (optional), skinned and washed**
- **1 head romaine lettuce leaves**
- **Salt, pepper, and lemon to taste**
- **Poppy seeds, for garnish (optional)**

In large pot, simmer Sonia's Basic Onion Formula at high temperature for 5 minutes.

Stir into the hot onion base: soybeans, chile, 1 cup of the corn, cilantro, tomatillos, romaine leaves, and 2 quarts of water. Bring to boil and simmer for one hour.

Let cool. Use a blender to puree cooled soup until smooth. (This can also be blended with a hand-held blender directly in the pot.)

Season to taste and add the reserved corn. Heat and serve.

fish

Biotin Tuna Surprise Salad/Sandwich

MAKES 4 SERVINGS

This tasty recipe fulfills the body's need for biotin, a deficiency of which may result in fatigue or depression. Serve this salad on a bed of greens and garnish with fresh mint or parsley (chewing parsley is good to take away the fishy taste), or garnish with cayenne pepper and fresh lemon slices. Alternatively, serve with whole wheat or corn tortillas, pita bread, or sheets of seaweed and red grapes.

1 6-ounce can tuna, drained

½ medium red onion, chopped

½ cup each chopped New Mexico green chile or any sweet pepper, chopped red cabbage, and yogurt cream (see directions below)

2 teaspoons flaxseeds, and toasted sesame seeds, or olive oil (optional)

1 teaspoon each curry powder, cinnamon, and cumin seeds

Pinch of sea salt

Mix all the ingredients together thoroughly.

Variations: Substitute 2 cups canned garbanzo (drained and pureed) for the tuna. Substitute ½ cup red grapes for the cabbage for a summery salad.

To make yogurt cream: *Place yogurt in a fine-mesh strainer, cover, and drain in the refrigerator overnight. Yogurt cream can be stored in the refrigerator for up to 1 week.*

MAKES 2 TO 4 SERVINGS

The trick to great risotto is stirring, stirring, stirring. This is a delicious meal for any day, and will impress guests (but—surprise—it is not difficult!)

> **3 tablespoons olive oil, divided**
> **I medium onion, diced**
> **2 medium tomatoes, finely chopped**
> **I cup mushroom**
> **I cup arborio rice**
> **I cup chicken broth, miso broth, or tomato juice**
> **I cup Marsala cooking wine, or any dry white wine, or an extra cup of broth**
> **I tablespoon butter**
> **2 to 3 cloves garlic, chopped**
> **2 cups shrimp (16 to 20 medium size, shells off)**

Sauté the onion, tomatoes, and mushrooms in 2 tablespoons of the oil over medium heat for 5 to 8 minutes, until soft.

Add the dry rice to the vegetables and "toast" for 2 minutes on high heat. Turn the heat back to medium.

Add the wine and continue cooking, stirring constantly. Once the wine is absorbed into the rice, add the broth and butter gradually, stirring constantly.

Sauté shrimp and minced garlic in the remaining olive oil, and serve over the risotto or on the side.

Variations: Use oysters instead of shrimp. Use I cup chopped fresh asparagus, green peas, or green soybeans instead of tomatoes.

snacks

Sonia's Strengthening Seed Snack

THIS RECIPE WILL MAKE ENOUGH FOR APPROXIMATELY 2 WEEKS

This is an excellent recipe for strengthening all your organs and hormones. One-half cup of this per week supplies your requirement for essential fatty acids and some phytohormonals through the spices and raisins.

> ⅓ **cup each (any ingredient can be optional) flaxseeds, sunflower seeds, black sesame seeds (can use white if black not available), anise seeds, fennel seeds, and raisins**

Mix everything together and store in tightly closed jar in cool, dry place. Eat about 1 to 2 tablespoons at a time throughout the day, or sprinkle on foods such as baked potatoes, cooked greens, salads, soups, cereals, yogurt, smoothies, and desserts such as pudding, fruit pies, and ice cream.

Yogurt Snack for Strong Immunity

MAKES 1½ CUPS

This recipe is designed to be therapeutic for cleansing, healing, and encouraging good bacteria. It is delicious, too. Snack on it anytime you have indigestion or an upset stomach.

> **1 cup low-fat yogurt**
> **2 to 4 cloves garlic, minced**
> **½ to 1 cup loosely packed chopped fresh mint or 1 tablespoon dried mint**

Mix all the ingredients together and refrigerate. Serve garnished with whole mint leaves, if desired.

Variation: *Top with flaxseeds for powerful cleansing and rejuvenating.*

Aged Garlic

Used therapeutically throughout Asia, the Mediterranean, and the Middle East, this is a delicacy to use on snack trays or to serve at parties. Aged garlic can last for as long as ten years.

2 pounds whole garlic bulbs
1 cup apple cider vinegar, or as needed
Pinch of salt

Choose a glass container with a lid (a jar works great). Place the garlic bulbs into the jar and fill with vinegar and salt. Cover the jar tightly and store in a dry, dark place. Do not refrigerate. You can keep this in your basement or garage or in a low cabinet that you seldom open.

Store for at least three months. Cultural wisdom teaches that the longer you keep it, the more therapeutic this delicacy becomes.

Serve as part of snack or dinner trays or as you would any condiment, such as pickles.

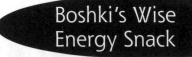

Boshki's Wise Energy Snack

This easy, healthy, and refreshing portable snack satisfies your desire for texture, color, and aroma for total wellness. Good for energy, PMS, mood swings, and insomnia.

Use any or all of the following:
½ cup mixed seeds, almonds, peanuts, walnuts, Brazil nuts, or pecans
a pinch of fennel seeds
1 cup mixed dried fruits: chopped apricots, figs, prunes, papaya, pineapple, raisins, dates, or crystallized ginger
2 cups mixed roasted garbanzo beans, soybeans, lentil, amaranth, wheat berries or roasted rice, granola, or other grain (see Roasted Garbanzos and Soybeans in chapter 6; that recipe can also be used for roasting lentils and grains)

Mix together all of the ingredients together in a glass jar, bowl, or freezer bag. This will stay fresh for weeks without refrigeration. You may top your cereal or yogurt (flavored or plain) or ricotta with this snack to make it a meal.

Variation: If you crave a lot of chocolate candy or cookies, adding a small amount of chocolate when you eat this means you'll eat less of the sweets, but still enjoy the taste.

sweet things

Saffron-Pumpkin Delight

SERVES 4

Aromatic, spicy, and colorful—this delightful recipe is perfect for after dinner or snacking and proves that rich-tasting desserts can be easy!

1 cup raisins
1 cup apple juice
3 apples (Rome red are good choice), cored and sliced
1 cup canned pumpkin or fresh pumpkin puree
½ teaspoon dried saffron
1 teaspoon each nutmeg, cinnamon, and pumpkin pie spice
½ cup each slivered almonds and chopped pumpkin seeds
Hibiscus leaves, fresh mint sprig, or berries, for garnish (optional)

Soak the raisins in the apple juice for 1 to 2 hours.
Preheat the oven to 350°F. Fold all the ingredients except the garnish together and pour into a glass baking dish.
Bake for 20 to 30 minutes. Garnish and serve warm.

Variations: Substitute peeled and sliced banana squash, yam, or sweet potato for the pumpkin. Use orange zest or shredded carrot instead of the saffron.

Yam Therapy for Hot Flashes

MAKES 4 TO 6 SERVINGS

Yams are a tasty, satisfying way to balance your hormones and get the bonus of beta-carotene, fiber, and vitamins A, C, and E.

1 cup canned crushed pineapple with juice
1 cup orange juice (from concentrate, or from 3 fresh oranges)
1 teaspoon cinnamon
1 tablespoon brown sugar
1 tablespoon olive or walnut oil
4 medium yams or sweet potatoes, scrubbed and cut into quarters
2 medium green apples, peeled and cut into quarters
½ cup slivered almonds
2 tablespoons sesame seeds, fennel seeds, cardamom seeds, or flaxseeds, for garnish (optional)

Preheat the oven to 350°F. Mix the crushed pineapple, orange juice, cinnamon, brown sugar, and oil in a small bowl. Set aside.
Place the yams and apples in a baking pan. Top with the juice mixture and almonds.
Bake for 25 to 40 minutes, or until tender. (If using a microwave, cook for 5 to 8 minutes.) Just before serving, sprinkle with the seeds.

Tonic Pears

SERVES 4 TO 6

Pears are used in Middle Eastern and Chinese medicine to balance the digestive tract for alkalinity and acidity. Ginger adds a slight flavor and aroma to the pears and may help to soothe the stomach. The pears can be served as dessert at brunch or dinner. Or serve this for breakfast.

> **4 ripe pears, halved and cored**
> **1-inch slice fresh ginger, peeled and minced**
> **Zest of 1 orange**
> **½ cup brown sugar or honey, or to taste**
> **20 cloves**
> **¼ cup walnut pieces or pecan pieces, toasted**

Preheat the oven to 375°F. Place the pears in a baking dish peel side down. Sprinkle the ginger, orange zest, and sugar over the pears.

Stick five cloves into each pear.

Cover and bake for 15 to 25 minutes (depending on size, variety of pears, and desired doneness).

When the pears are soft and turning mushy, take them out and drizzle juice from the pan over the pears. Top with roasted walnuts or pecans and serve.

Variations: *Top with yogurt just before serving for added protein. Garnish with fresh mint and dried berries for additional flavor. Add 1 teaspoon powdered licorice root (available in health food stores) instead of sugar or honey for more phytohormonal benefits.*

References

American Institute for Cancer Research. 2001. Cancer researchers warn about obesity-cancer link. October 11. http://www.charitywire.com/charity10/00256.html.

Beck, B, A. Burlet, J. P. Max, and A. Stricher-Krongrad. 2000. Neuropeptide Y, plasma leptin and body weight gain and composition. *Food Drug Law Journal* 55(3):389–433.

Bell, S. J., and G. K. Goodrick. 2002. A functional food product for the management of weight. *Critical Reviews in Food Science and Nutrition* 42(2): 163–78.

Brody, J. 1998. Study challenges idea of PMS as emotional disorder. *New York Times*, January 22, A1.

Callaway, C. W. 1987. Obesity. *Public Health Reports* July-August Suppl.:26–9.

Carper, J. 1988. *The Food Pharmacy*. New York: Bantam Doubleday Dell.

Chen, W. F., M. H. Huang, C. H. Tzang, M. Yang, and M. S. Wong. 2003. Inhibitory actions of genistein in human breast cancer (MCF-7) cells. *Biochimica et Biophysica Acta.* 1638(2):187–96.

Childers, J. M., J. Chu, L. F. Voigt, P. Feigl, H. K. Tamimi, E. W. Franklin, D. S. Alberts, and F. L. Meyskens Jr. 1995. Chemoprevention of cervical cancer with folic acid: A phase III Southwest Oncology Group Intergroup study. *Cancer Epidemiology, Biomarkers and Prevention* 4(2):155–9.

Cimons M. 1997. As obesity standard drops, dieters' spirits may follow. *Los Angeles Times* June 5, A16.

Clayman H. M., and N. S. Jaffe. 1988. Spontaneous enlargement of neodymium: YAG posterior capsulotomy in aphakic and pseudophakic patients. *Journal of Cataract and Refractive Surgery* 14(6):667–9.

Cowan, L. D., L. Gordis, J. A. Tonascia, and G. S. Jones. 1981. Breast cancer incidence in women with a history of progesterone deficiency. *American Journal of Epidemiology* 114(2):209–17.

Dharmananda, S. 1998. Countering the side effects of modern medical therapies with Chinese herbs. http://www.itmonline.org/arts/sidefx. htm.

Feskanich, D., V. Singh, W. C. Willett, and G. A. Colditz. 2002. Vitamin A intake and hip fractures among postmenopausal women. *JAMA* 287(1): 47–54.

Fujiki, H., M. Suganuma, M. Kurus, S. Okabe, Y. Imayoshi, and T. Taniguchi Yoshida. 2003. TNF-alpha releasing inhibitors as cancer preventive agents from traditional herbal medine and combination cancer preventive agents from traditional herbal medicine and combination cancer prevention study with EGCG and sulindac or tamoxifen. *Mutation Research* 523–524:119–25.

Gaemi-Hashemi, S., J. A. Clark, and S. Margen. 1998. The benefit of combining Western and Eastern food models on women's hormonal balance. A talk given at San Francisco State University. (Abstract: American Dietetics Association, vol. 98, 9-A25)

Gaemi-Hashemi S. 1992. Attitudes and practices toward breastfeeding among Persian and Asian immigrant women. *Journal of the American Dietetic Association* 92:354–5.

Genet, J. 1995. Natural remedies for vaginal infections. *Sidahora* (Winter): 40–1.

Ghaemi, Hashemi S. 1980. Acculturation of food habits and attitude of Iranian and Iranian-American. Master's thesis, San Francisco State University. California.

Ghaemi S., and J. A. Clarke. 1990. A complete new lifetime multicultural solution for weight control and wellness *Journal of the American Dietetic Association* 9:A-20.

Gordon, D. 1998–1999. You are what you eat: Dr. John Glaspy proves diet can alter breast issue. *UCLA Cancer Discoveries Magazine.* http://www.cancer.mednet.ucla.edu/discoveries/1998/drglaspy.html.

Grisolia, S. 1974. Hypoxia, saffron, and cardiovascular disease. *Lancet* 2(7871):41–2.

Heaney R. P., K. M. Davies, and M. J. Barger-Lux. 2002. Calcium and weight: Clinical studies. *Journal of the American College of Nutrition* 21(2):152S–155S.

Infeld, K., C. Ebersold, Z. Haydar, K. Stewart, and J. Fleg. 1997. Exercise improves heart function in elderly people with heart failure. http://www.hopkinsmedicine.org/press/1997/november/971107.htm.

Ingels, D. 2002. Cranberry juice may prevent urinary tract infections. *Healthnotes Newswire* July 18.

Karter, A. J., E. J. Mayer-Davis, J. V. Selby, R. P. D'Agostino Jr, S. M. Haffner, P. Sholinsky, R. Bergman, M. F. Saad, and R. F. Hamman. 1996. Insulin sensitivity and abdominal obesity in African-American, Hispanic, and non-Hispanic white men and women. *Diabetes.* 45(11):1547–55.

Katsouyanni, K., W. Willett, D. Trichopoulos, P. Boyle, A. Trichopoulou, S. Vasilaros, J. Papadiamantis, and B. MacMahon. 1988. Risk of breast cancer among Greek women in relation to nutrient intake. *Cancer* 61(1): 181–5.

Lamendola C. 2003. Early and more vigorous detection of diabetes. *Journal of Cardiovascular Nursing* 18(2):103–7

Lang, D. A., D. R. Matthews, M. Burnett, and R. C. Turner. 1997. Brief, irregular oscillations of basal plasma insulin and glucose concentrations in diabetic man. *Diabetes* 30(5):435–9.

Lean, M. E. 2000. Obesity: Burdens of illness and strategies for prevention or management. *Drugs Today (Barc)* 36(11):773–84.

Lemann, J., Jr., J. A. Pleuss, and R. W. Gray. 1993. Potassium causes calcium retention in healthy adults. *The Journal of Nutrition* 123(9):1623–6.

Ley, R. 1999. The modification of breathing behavior. Pavlovian and operant control in emotion and cognition. *Behavior Modification* 23(3):441–79.

Lichenstein, A. H. 2003. Dietary fat and cardiovascular disease risk: Quantity or quality? *Journal of Women's Health* 12(2):109–14.

Liu, J., J. E. Burdette, H. Xu, C. Gu, R. B. van Breemen, K. P. Bhat, N. Booth, A. I. Constantinou, J. M. Pezzuto, H. H. Fong, N. R. Farnsworth, and J. L. Bolton. 2001. Evaluation of estrogenic activity of plant extracts for the potential treatment of menopausal symptoms. *Journal of Agriculture and Food Chemistry* 49(5):2472–9.

Ludwig, D. 2002. The glycemic index. *Journal of the American Medical Associates* 287:2414–2423

Manon, R. R., R. Patel, T. Zhang, D. Henderson, W. Tome, J. Fenwick, B. Paliwal, and M. Mehta. 2003. CT-based analysis of free-breathing vs. maximum inspiratory breath hold techniques for 3-D conformal radiation therapy and intensity modulated radiation therapy in lung cancer: A potential basis for dose-escalation. *International Journal of Radiation Oncology, Biology, Physics* 57(2 Suppl.):S417.

Marckmann, P. 2003. Fishing for heart protection. *The American Journal of Clinical Nutrition* 78(1):1–2.

Margen, S. 1992. *The Wellness Encyclopedia of Food and Nutrition: How to Buy, Store, and Prepare Every Variety of Fresh Food.* New York: Rebus, Inc.

Marx, J. J. M. 1999. Iron, atherosclerosis, and ischemic heart disease. *Archives of Internal Medicine* 159:1542–8.

Mayo Clinic. 1998. Fish and heart health: Make fish a regular on your plate. *Mayo Clinic Health Letter* (July).

McConnaughey, J. 2003. One in three U.S. children at risk for diabetes. *Associated Press International,* June 16.

McEwen, B. S. 1998. Excitotoxicity, stress hormones and the aging nervous system. *Integrative Medicine* 1:135–41.

Mertz, W. 1993. Chromium in human nutrition: A review. *The Journal of Nutrition* 123(4):626–33.

Michalkiewicz, M., K. M. Knestaut, E. Y. Bytchkova, and T. Michalkiewicz. 2003. Hypotension and reduced catecholamines in neuropeptide Y transgenic rats. *Hypertension* 41(5):1056–62.

Miller, C. J., E. V. Dunn, and I. B. Hashim. 2003. The glycaemic index of dates and date/yoghurt mixed meals. Are dates 'the candy that grows on trees'. *European Journal of Clinical Nutrition* 57(3):427–30.

Muti, P., H. L. Bradlow, A. Micheli, V. Krogh, J. L. Freudenheim, H. J. Schunemann, M. Stanulla, J. Yang, D. W. Sepkovic, M. Trevisan, and F. Berrino. 2000. Estrogen metabolism and risk of breast cancer: A prospective study of the 2:16alpha-hydroxyestrone ratio in premenopausal and postmenopausal women. *Epidemiology* 11(6):635–40.

Nakamura, Y., N. Kawamoto, Y. Ohto, K. Torikai, A. Murakami, and H. Ohigashi. 1999. A diacetylenic spiroketal enol ether epoxide, AL-1, from *Artemisia lactiflora* inhibits 12-O-tetradecanoylphorbol-13-acetate- induced tumor promotion possibly by suppression of oxidative stress. *Cancer Letters* 140(1-2): 37–45.

Newcomb, P. A., B. E. Storer, M. Longnecker, R. Mittendorf, E. R. Greenberg, R. W. Clapp, K. Burke, W. Willett, and B. MacMahon. 1994. Lactation and a reduced risk of premenopausal breast cancer. *The New English Journal of Medicine* 330(2):81–87.

Olsson, H., A. Borg, M. Ferno, T. R. Moller, and J. Ranstam. 1991. Early oral contraceptive use and premenopausal breast cancer—a review of studies performed in southern Sweden. *Cancer Detection and Prevention* 15(4): 265–71.

Ostman, E. M., H. G. L. Elmstahl, and I. M. Bjorck. 2001. Inconsistency between glycemic and insulinemic responses to regular and fermented milk products. *The American Journal of Clinical Nutrition.* 74(1):96–100.

Pandey, D. K., R. Shekelle, B. J. Selwyn, C. Tangney, and J. Stamler. 1995. Dietary vitamin C and beta-carotene and risk of death in middle-aged men. *American Journal of Epidemiology* 142(12):1269–78.

Polk M. 2002. Herbs and Spices that Reduce Cancer Risk. International Research Conference on Food, Nutrition and Cancer, American Institute for Cancer Research, July 11, Washington, DC.

Rao, A. V., and S. Agarwal. 2000. Role of antioxidant lycopene in cancer and heart disease. *Journal of the American College of Nutrition* 19(5): 563–9.

Rowland, I. R., H. Wiseman, T. A. Sanders, H. Adlercreutz, and E. A. Bowey. 2000. Interindividual variation in metabolism of soy isoflavones and lignans: Influence of habitual diet on equal production by the gut microflora. *Nutrition and Cancer* 36(1):27–32.

Sellers, T. A., L. H. Kushi, J. R. Cerhan, R. A. Vierkant, S. M. Gapstur, C. M. Vachon, J. E. Olson, T. M. Therneau, and A. R. Folsom. 2001. Dietary folate intake, alcohol, and risk of breast cancer in a prospective study of postmenopausal women. *Epidemiology* 12(4):420–8.

Severson, K. 2003. Obesity "a threat" to U.S. security: Surgeon general urges cultural shift in eating habits. *San Francisco Chronicle*, January 7, A1.

Sherman, P. W., and J. Billings. 1998. Antimicrobial functions of spice use: Why some like it hot. *Quarterly Review of Biology* 73(1):3–49.

Siddiqui, M. T., and M. Siddiqui. 1976. Hypolipidemic principles of *Cicer arietinum*: Biochanin-A and formononetin. *Lipids* 1:243–6.

Spicer, D., D. Shoupe, and M. Pike. 1991. Gonadotropin-releasing hormone agonist plus add-back sex steroids to reduce risk of breast cancer. *Journal of the National Cancer Institute* 83:1763.

Steinmetz, K. A., and J. D. Potter. 1996. Vegetables, fruit, and cancer prevention: A review. *Journal of the American Dietetic Association* 96 (10):1027–39.

Taylor, S. E. 2003. Letter in response to health claim petition—walnuts and coronary heart disease (Docket No. 02P-0292), July 14. Office of Nutritional Products, Labeling and Dietary Supplements, Center for Food Safety and Applied Nutrition. Washington, D.C.

Teuscher, T., P. Baillod, J. B. Rosman, and A. Teuscher. 1987. Absence of diabetes in a rural West African population with a high carbohydrate/cassava diet. *Lancet* 1(8536):765–8.

Tokudome S., T. Nagaya, H. Okuyama, Y. Tokudome, N. Imaeda, I. Kitagawa, N. Fujiwara, M. Ikeda, C. Goto, H. Ichikawa, K. Kuriki, K. Takekuma, A. Shimoda, K. Hirose, and T. Usui. 2000. Japanese versus Mediterranean diets and cancer. *Asian Pacific Journal of Cancer Prevention* 1(1):61–66.

Toobert, D. J., L. A. Strycker, and R. E. Glasgow. 2002. Lifestyle change in women with coronary heart disease: What do we know? *Journal of Women's Health* 7(6):685–99.

Walis, A., J. Bratosiewicz, B. Sikorska, P. Brown, D. C. Gajdusek, and P. P. Liberski. 2003. Ultrastructural changes in the optic nerves of rodents with experimental Creutzfeldt-Jakob disease (CJD), Gerstmann-Straussler-Scheinker disease (GSS) or scrapie. *Journal of Comparative Pathology* 129(2–3):213–25.

Zava, D., C. M. Dollbaum, and M. Blen. 1988. Estrogen and progestin bioactivity of foods, herbs, and spices. *Proceedings of the Society for Experimental Biology and Medicine* 217(3):369–78.

Zava, D., and G. Duwe. Estrogenic and antiproliferative properties of genistein and other flavonoids in human breast cancer cells in vitro: *Nutrition and Cancer* 27(1):31–40.

Zeml, in press

Some Other
New Harbinger Titles

Eating Mindfully, Item 3503, $13.95

Living with RSDS, Item 3554 $16.95

The Ten Hidden Barriers to Weight Loss, Item 3244 $11.95

The Sjogren's Syndrome Survival Guide, Item 3562 $15.95

Stop Feeling Tired, Item 3139 $14.95

Responsible Drinking, Item 2949 $18.95

The Mitral Valve Prolapse/Dysautonomia Survival Guide, Item 3031 $14.95

Stop Worrying Abour Your Health, Item 285X $14.95

The Vulvodynia Survival Guide, Item 2914 $15.95

The Multifidus Back Pain Solution, Item 2787 $12.95

Move Your Body, Tone Your Mood, Item 2752 $17.95

The Chronic Illness Workbook, Item 2647 $16.95

Coping with Crohn's Disease, Item 2655 $15.95

The Woman's Book of Sleep, Item 2493 $14.95

The Trigger Point Therapy Workbook, Item 2507 $19.95

Fibromyalgia and Chronic Myofascial Pain Syndrome, second edition, Item 2388 $19.95

Kill the Craving, Item 237X $18.95

Rosacea, Item 2248 $13.95

Thinking Pregnant, Item 2302 $13.95

Shy Bladder Syndrome, Item 2272 $13.95

Help for Hairpullers, Item 2329 $13.95

Coping with Chronic Fatigue Syndrome, Item 0199 $13.95

The Stop Smoking Workbook, Item 0377 $17.95

Multiple Chemical Sensitivity, Item 173X $16.95

Call **toll free, 1-800-748-6273,** or log on to our online bookstore at **www.newharbinger.com** to order. Have your Visa or Mastercard number ready. Or send a check for the titles you want to New Harbinger Publications, Inc., 5674 Shattuck Ave., Oakland, CA 94609. Include $4.50 for the first book and 75¢ for each additional book, to cover shipping and handling. (California residents please include appropriate sales tax.) Allow two to five weeks for delivery.

Prices subject to change without notice.

Breaking the Bonds of Irritable Bowel Syndrome, Item 1888 $14.95